María del Pilar Díaz Martínez

Pain management in physiotherapy using dry needling

María del Pilar Díaz Martínez

Pain management in physiotherapy using dry needling

Lower limb

ScienciaScripts

Imprint

Cover image: www.ingimage.com

This book is a translation from the original published under ISBN 978-613-9-43418-3.

Publisher:
Sciencia Scripts
is a trademark of
Dodo Books Indian Ocean Ltd. and OmniScriptum S.R.L publishing group

120 High Road, East Finchley, London, N2 9ED, United Kingdom
Str. Armeneasca 28/1, office 1, Chisinau MD-2012, Republic of Moldova, Europe
Printed at: see last page
ISBN: 978-620-8-29318-5

Table of Contents

1. INTRODUCTION TO DRY NEEDLING (PS).

Dry needling (SP) is a therapeutic technique that has gained a prominent place in the field of physical therapy, but its application requires a deep anatomical knowledge and specific precautions to ensure patient safety (1, 2).

First of all, it is essential to consider the risks associated with this technique. Dry needling, if not performed correctly, can lead to complications such as pneumothorax, injury to blood vessels, nerves or even internal organs. It is therefore essential that the physical therapist has a clear command of human anatomy, especially the structures to be avoided during puncture (3, 4).

Structures to avoid include the pleura and lungs, as a deep puncture in these areas could cause a pneumothorax. It is also crucial to be alert to the presence of blood vessels, avoiding punctures in veins, and to nerve injuries, which may cause electrical pain on contact with the needle. If this sensation is felt, the needle should be repositioned immediately to avoid damage. In addition, care should be taken with internal organs, such as the kidney, and joints, where an inappropriate puncture could result in serious complications (5, 6).

The effectiveness of dry needling depends largely on accurate diagnosis of myofascial trigger points. Evidence supports its use in a variety of musculoskeletal conditions, making it a valuable tool for treating conditions such as myofascial pain, shoulder pain associated with hemiparesis or impingement, chronic low back and neck pain, as well as headaches and migraines. It is also used in cases of nerve entrapment syndromes, such as carpal tunnel, and in the treatment of tendinopathies and plantar fasciitis. However, dry needling is not without precautions. One of the most common effects is pain, which can be intense, but is usually temporary. It is essential to follow proper needle-handling techniques, as there is a risk of bending or breaking the needles during the procedure. Pneumothorax, although rare, is a major concern; therefore, deep chest puncture should be avoided (7, 8).

Vascular lesions are another risk to consider. Therefore, knowledge of vascular anatomy is vital to prevent bleeding. In the event of bleeding, pressure should be applied immediately. Nerve and visceral injuries are also significant concerns. For this reason, it is essential to be familiar with the anatomy of the peripheral and central nerves, as well as the location of internal organs, to avoid damage. The risk of infection must also be taken into account. It is crucial to follow strict aseptic protocols, using sterile needles and ensuring proper waste management. In addition, vegetative reactions such as vasovagal syncope are common. To prevent fainting, it is advisable to perform the puncture while the patient is in decubitus (9, 10, 11).

PS is an invasive procedure used in physical therapy to treat pain and muscle dysfunction, but it carries certain risks that require careful patient evaluation. There are absolute contraindications, such as needle phobia, patient refusal, inability to give consent, medical emergencies, and areas with lymphedema. Relative contraindications are also identified, such as bleeding tendency, immune system compromises, vascular disease, diabetes and pregnancy. It is crucial that the clinician perform a detailed analysis before proceeding. In addition, special precautions should be taken into account for vulnerable groups, such as children and patients with conditions such as epilepsy or anxiety (12, 13).

Safety in the practice of SP is fundamental. Procedures are classified into superficial dry needling (SDP) and trigger point dry needling (TPD), each with its own risks. Adverse effects can range from bruising and local pain to more serious complications, although these are rare. Although the literature has not yet fully explored these risks, clinical experience indicates that most adverse effects are mild and reversible. To prevent infection, hand hygiene is essential. Practitioners should follow prevention guidelines that address the chain of infection, which includes the infectious agent, the reservoir, the exit and entry port, as well as the susceptible host. Hygiene measures include hand washing with appropriate soap, glove use, and puncture site preparation. The choice of hand hygiene products should consider their skin irritant potential. Gloves are mandatory to prevent contact with body fluids, and care should be taken when handling them to avoid puncture injuries. In case of an accident, the wound should be washed immediately and medical attention sought (14, 15, 16, 17, 18).

During the procedure, effective communication with the patient is key. Post-treatment discomfort is common, and it is vital to inform the patient about it to reduce anxiety. If the patient experiences acute pain or any worrisome symptoms, the clinician should act immediately, removing the needle and applying the necessary measures (19).

2. METHODS OF PS.

Dry needling (DP) is a method used to treat myofascial trigger points (MTrPs) and is classified into several modalities, depending on factors such as the tool used, the depth of needle insertion and the therapeutic approach of the practitioner. The main categories are superficial dry needling (SDP) and deep dry needling (DSP) (20, 21, 22).

In PSS, such as the Peter Baldry technique, the needle is inserted into the subcutaneous tissues without reaching the PGM, and its effectiveness is based on the reduction of pain and associated hyperalgesia. Another technique in this category is Fu's subcutaneous puncture, which mobilizes the needle into the subcutaneous tissue at a distance from the PGM. In both, the duration of insertion and stimulation can be adjusted according to the patient's response. On the other hand, PSP focuses on the PGMs and uses techniques such as Hong's rapid entry and exit, which seeks to elicit local twitch responses by rapidly inserting and withdrawing the needle. Another technique, Gunn's intramuscular stimulation, treats chronic pain by rapidly manipulating the needle to release endorphins and relieve pain. Dry electropuncture, which uses electrical current, is also notable for its proposed mechanisms that induce muscle contractions, facilitating the elimination of pain-sensitizing substances (23, 24, 25).

Both dry needling modalities, PSS and PSP, have different mechanisms of action. In PSS, stimulation of A-beta nerve fibers helps block pain transmission, while PSP induces a "washout" of pain-perpetuating substances and improves pH in the area of the PGM, which may normalize its function. In addition, PSP has been observed to improve oxygenation and blood flow, which counteracts the hypoxia typical of PGMs. PSP also impacts connective tissue and muscle fascia. The needles used are fine, allowing specific interaction with the tissue. As the needle is rotated, a "ball" of collagen is created that generates stretch in the subcutaneous and intermuscular layers. This causes viscoelastic responses in the tissue, which can lead to collagen relaxation and reorganization (26, 27, 28, 29).

Fascia, composed of dense, lax connective tissue, plays a crucial role in myofascial pain. Restrictions in the fascia, especially in the perimysium, may contribute to the formation of tight bands that generate pain. Although there is a clear connection between fascia and PGMs, research on how dry needling affects these structures is limited. There is an urgent need for studies that explore these interactions to better understand myofascial pain and optimize therapeutic interventions (30, 31, 32, 33).

3. PROTOCOL FOR A CORRECT PRACTICAL APPLICATION IN PS.

Dry needling is a technique that requires careful and methodical attention to ensure its efficacy and safety. The process begins with the collection of the medical history, where the physical therapist collects detailed information about the patient's medical history, current symptoms and performs a thorough physical assessment. This allows the trigger points to be properly identified and the appropriate intervention to be chosen (34, 35).

Once the information has been gathered, the next step is to inform the patient about the proposed treatment. This includes explaining the dry needling technique, its benefits and possible risks. It is essential that the patient understands the procedure and signs an informed consent, which not only protects the physical therapist, but also establishes a relationship of trust. Hygiene is another critical aspect. Before starting the puncture, the physical therapist should wash his or her hands and disinfect the patient's skin to avoid infection. In addition, correct positioning of the patient in a comfortable position is essential to facilitate access to the area to be treated and ensure that the procedure is performed effectively. Before the puncture is performed, the diagnosis and location of the muscle trigger point (MTP) must be confirmed. This step is vital for the treatment to be specific and effective. During the execution of the puncture, it is important that the physical therapist acts with skill and maintains constant communication with the patient, adjusting the technique according to his or her comfort (36, 37, 38).

Once the puncture is completed, certain post-procedural care must be followed. This includes hemostasis techniques to control any bleeding and provide instructions on the care of the treated area. Scheduling a follow-up is essential to assess the efficacy of the treatment and to address possible side effects (39, 40) .

Dry needling is used to treat myofascial pain syndrome, which involves the release of acetylcholine and the formation of trigger points. Although it is intended to relieve pain, the technique can cause injury to muscle and nerve fibers. The needles used are larger than the muscle fibers themselves, resulting in lacerations (41, 42).

Muscle injury initiates an inflammatory process that activates immune cells responsible for clearing cellular debris and promoting regeneration. As the satellite cells are activated and become myoblasts, they begin to repair the damaged muscle fiber, a process that can take about seven days. In addition, dry needling can cause damage to the axons, leading to degeneration of the distal segment. However, the inflammatory response aids in the removal of debris and promotes axonal growth to restore function. Although complications may arise, studies show that, in general, muscle regeneration and reinnervation occur effectively, demonstrating the reparative potential of the technique (43, 44).

4. NON-MYOFASCIAL TRIGGER POINTS (NMTPS).

Dry needling (DP) is a therapeutic technique that consists of inserting needles through the skin without administering medication, mainly used to treat non-myofascial trigger points (NMTPs). These points are identified as painful areas that do not correspond to myofascial trigger points (MTrPs) and may include tendon attachment areas, sheaths, fasciae, and subcutaneous tissues (45).

PGNMs can be provoked by local spasms derived from the activation of a PGM. Hong defines them as foci of sensitization where nociceptors are hyperstimulated, allowing PS to produce pain relief, even using acupuncture points. Traditional Chinese acupuncture is one of the first techniques applied to PGNMs, and other techniques can be used, such as PS with multiple rapid insertions, which seeks to desensitize nociceptors, or PS for soft tissue release, which relieves tension in muscles and tissues (46, 47).

The mechanisms that account for pain relief by PS include activation of the pain inhibitory system, interruption of the PGM cycle, and stimulation of nociceptors, which interrupts the pain signal. To apply PS effectively, it is important to properly choose the type of needle and follow a precise insertion technique. After the procedure, compression should be applied to the treated area to minimize pain (48, 49).

The most prominent techniques are rapid entry and exit with rotation, ideal for patients with fibromyalgia, and PS for soft tissue release, which uses cannulas to inject substances that facilitate the release of tissue adhesions. These methodologies allow effective treatment of PGNMs, achieving significant pain relief and tension release in tendons and ligaments (50).

5. CLASSIFICATION AND PS IN THE PGM OF THE DIFFERENT MUSCULATURE.

5.1. PS for thoracic musculature.

5.1.1. Anterior serratus.

- Location of PG: They are usually found between the fifth and sixth ribs. They can also be located in the midline of the muscle fibers on the ventral aspect of the muscle and on the vertebral border of the scapula. This muscle is essential for shoulder function and, therefore, PGMs in it can affect mobility and cause pain (51, 52).
- Pain referred by the serratus anterior PGMs frequently manifests in the thorax, where the PGMs are located. It can also be found medial to the inferior angle of the scapula. In less common cases, the pain may extend to the medial aspect of the arm, reaching the wrist and hand. The pain may be persistent and show little variation with postural changes. Although the serratus anterior is not a primary inspiratory muscle, PGMs in it may be related to respiratory difficulties and chest pain associated with myocardial infarction, in combination with the pectoralis major (51, 52).
- Associated symptoms: oppressive chest pain, often accompanied by anxiety in the patient and weakness and alteration in the pattern of muscle activation, especially in activities that require arm elevation (51, 52).
- Activation mechanisms (51, 52):
    - Direct Mechanisms:
        - Chronic overload: Activities that involve keeping the arms elevated or performing repetitive movements, such as manual labor or certain sports.
        - Intense exercise: Activities such as push-ups, which can result in overload.
    - Indirect Mechanisms:
        - Joint dysfunctions: Problems in the shoulder joint (glenohumeral, sternoclavicular, acromioclavicular) may contribute to serratus anterior weakness.

    - Cervical Spine: Alterations in the cervical spine can cause a delay in the activation of the serratus anterior, which can increase the load on the cervical and thoracic structures.
    - Radiculopathy: Compression of peripheral nerves can activate PGMs.
    - Other muscles, such as the scalenes, iliocostalis thoracis and diaphragm, may influence the activation of serratus anterior PGMs.
- PS (51, 52):
  - Patient Position: Position in lateral decubitus, with the affected side up.
  - Location of the PGM:
    - Place the patient's arm in extension, which causes adduction of the scapula, allowing the lateral fibers of the serratus anterior to become more accessible.
    - Flex the elbow to approximately 90 degrees and rest the hand on the iliac crest.
    - Palpate transversely to locate the PGM, which is usually in the mid-axillary line above the fifth and sixth ribs.
  - Needle: Use a 0.25 mm x 25 mm needle, avoiding longer needles that can reach the lung.
  - Puncture technique:
    - Fasten the band taut with two fingers, leaving the PGM between them.
    - Slide your fingers over or under the taut band to open up space.
    - Insert the needle tangentially to the thorax.
- Dangers and precautions: The risk of pneumothorax although the technique is unlikely to reach the lung, caution should be exercised to avoid complications such as pneumothorax (51, 52).

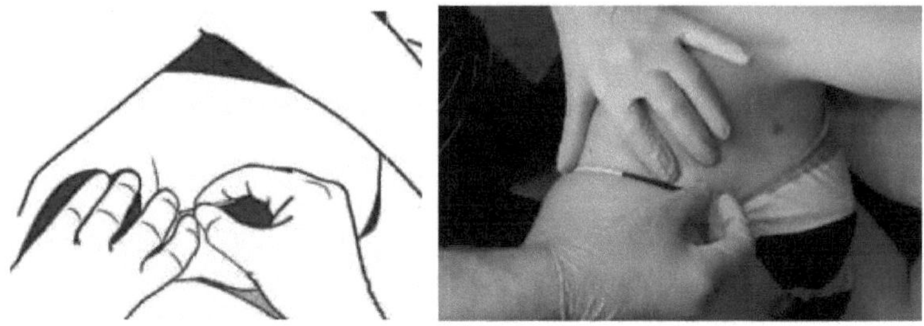

Figure 1. PS in PGM of the serratus anterior (53, 54).

5.1.2. Postero-superior serratus.

- Location and characteristics of MTrPs: Myofascial trigger points of the serratus posterosuperioris muscle are usually located in the central part of the muscle, just medial to the vertebral border of the superior angle of the scapula. According to Simons et al, PGMs can be identified at the costal insertion of the muscle, representing insertional entities (enthesopathies). They point out the insertions at the level of the fourth rib as the cause of what they call scapulocostal syndrome (55, 56).
- Referred pain pattern: The referred pain pattern usually coincides with the area medial to the superior angle of the scapula, accompanied by pain in the posterior area of the shoulder and arm, being more intense in the shoulder and elbow. The pain may extend to the ulnar side of the forearm and hand, which leads to the patient being frequently diagnosed with cervicobrachialgia or cervical radiculopathy. Pain may also be present in the pectoral region, projecting forward from the superior angle of the scapula, crossing the lung. Sometimes, PGMs can cause symptoms of a painful, stiff neck, with difficulty in homolateral rotation. This reaction, although unusual, may be explained by the proprioceptive function of the muscle, which has a high density of muscle spindles (55, 56).

- Clinical: Deep persistent pain in the upper part of the scapula, with little variability. Associated pain along the upper extremity (55, 56).
- Activation mechanisms: Activation of the PGMs of the serratus posterosuperioris can occur directly due to episodes of prolonged coughing and respiratory problems that overload the accessory inspiratory musculature, as well as by postures and activities involving the use of the upper limb, where the scapula exerts pressure on the muscle. These PGMs may coexist with those of other muscles, such as the medial trapezius, rhomboids, thoracic iliocostalis, levator scapulae or scalenes, and may be activated indirectly by these muscles when referring pain in their area (55, 56).
- Related muscles: scalenes, rhomboids, medial trapezius, iliocostalis, levator scapulae (55, 56).
- PS (55, 56):
    - Lancing technique: The patient is placed in prone position with the hand on the affected side behind the back, allowing internal rotation of the humerus and anteriorization of the shoulder. This helps to separate the internal border of the scapula, displacing the superior angle upward and outward, slightly stretching the trapezius and rhomboid muscles overlying the serratus. To locate the PGMs, deep palpation is performed against the ribs in the area, where taut bands can often be detected. The direction of the fibers of the serratus posterosuperioris and rhomboids is oblique, unlike the trapezius, which has a more horizontal direction. To distinguish between the two, first identify the taut band with the patient's arm along the body. By asking the patient to place the hand behind the back, the fibers of the rhomboids are displaced, which helps to identify whether the band corresponds to the serratus posterosuperioris.
    - Position: Prone position with the hand behind the back.
    - Needle size: 0.25 mm x 25 mm.

- Precautions: Avoid pneumothorax. In case the PGM is identified, the band is fixed with two fingers, and the needle is inserted medial to the finger fixing the PGM, trying to go through it with a tangential approach to the thorax to avoid reaching the lung. In most cases, it is recommended to use a 0.25 mm x 25 mm needle.

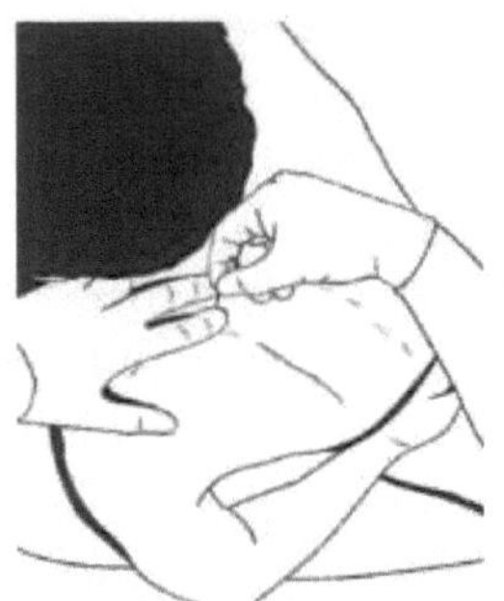
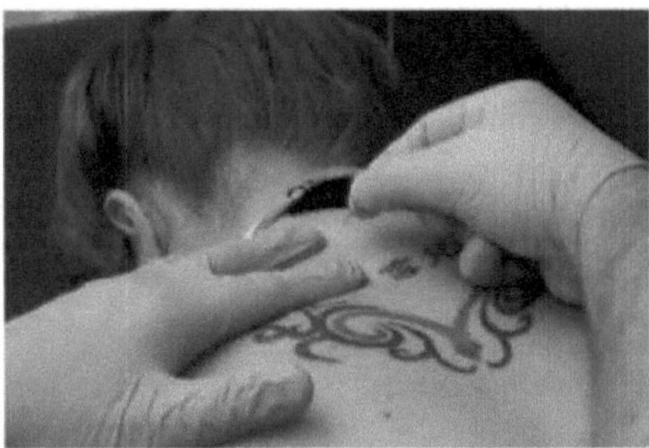

Figure 2. PS in PGM for serratus postero-superior (53, 54).

- Dangers and precautions: The main risk during this procedure is pneumothorax, so it is crucial to be careful when puncturing the affected area.

5.1.3. Posterior-inferior serratus.

- Location and characteristics of the PGMs of the serratus posteroinferioris: They can be found in the thoracolumbar area, outside the iliocostalis, above the last ribs. This muscle is less known, and the literature describing its possible symptomatology is quite limited (51, 52, 55, 56).
- Referred pain pattern: The referred pain pattern is located just above the muscle, usually adding to a compound pattern that includes other muscles and structures, often presenting in low back pain. PGMs of the serratus posteroinferioris often coexist with PGMs of the erector spinae. When this muscle is the source of pain,

the patient tends to describe a stabbing pain, not very intense, but annoying and persistent, with slight mechanical variability, without significant changes during inspiration or forced expiration. This condition may occur after other causes of pain have been treated, when the patient has achieved improvement, but still experiences residual pain (51, 52, 55, 56).

- Clinical (51, 52, 55, 56):
  - Pain: stabbing, with slight mechanical variability.
  - Residual pain: persists after treating other causes of low back pain.
- Related muscles: Longissimus thoracis, iliocostalis thoracis and latissimus dorsi (51, 52, 55, 56).
- PS (51, 52, 55, 56):
  - Lancing technique: The patient should be positioned in prone decubitus. Once the thoracolumbar hinge is located, look for the tense band and the PGM, palpating obliquely outside the iliocostal and against the firm base of the last ribs. The latissimus dorsi fibers at this level have an oblique, more vertical direction, while the direction of the iliocostalis is markedly vertical. It is recommended to use a 0.25 mm x 25 mm needle in most patients, avoiding longer needles that could increase the risk of pneumothorax.
  - To perform the puncture:
    - Localization: Fix the taut band with two fingers placed on both sides of the PGM, trying to locate it over the rib.
    - Direction of the needle: Since the fibers are in oblique relation to the ribs, the fingertips holding the band are likely to be in the intercostal spaces, reducing the risk of pneumothorax.
    - Insertion technique: For greater safety, the fingers should slide under the band, allowing the needle to be inserted as tangential as possible to the thorax.

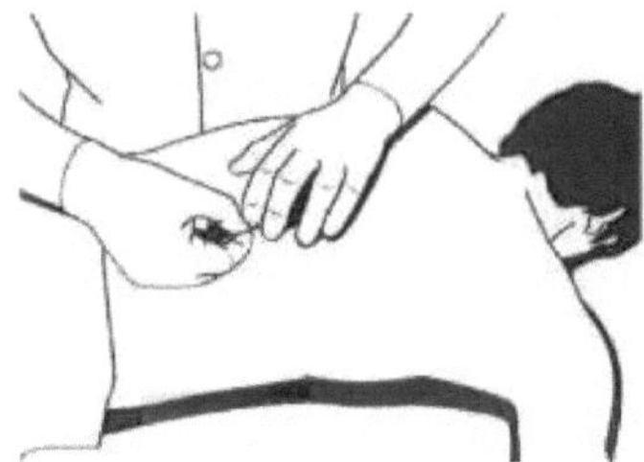
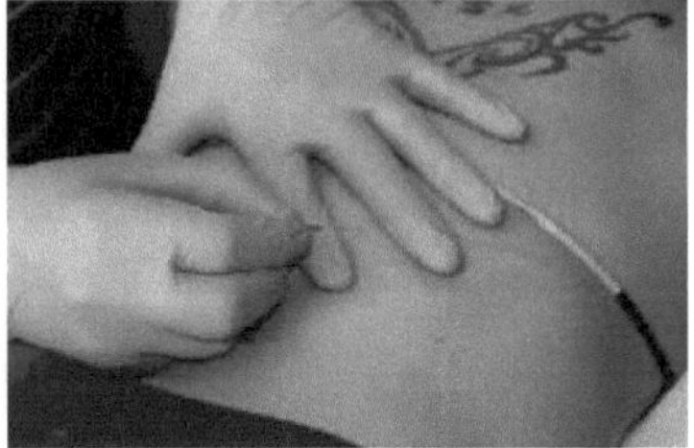

Figure 3. PS in PGM for serratus posterior-inferior (53, 54).

- Hazards and precautions: Risk of pneumothorax, the main concern is to prevent the needle from reaching the lung during puncture (51, 52, 55, 56).

5.1.4. Pectoralis major.

Myofascial trigger points (MTrPs) in the pectoralis major are distributed in several areas, and each of these areas is associated with specific patterns of referred pain. The different divisions of the muscle and their clinical implications are described below (57, 58).

- Localization and pain patterns (57, 58):
  - Clavicular portion:
    - Referred pain: Mainly in the anterior aspect of the shoulder, although local pain may be referred.
    - Description: The PGMs of this portion are usually located in the upper part of the muscle.
  - Sternocostal division:
    - Location of PGMs: They are generally located in the central part of their fibers.
    - Referred pain: It may include pain that extends through the anterior part of the thorax and below the medial epicondyle in the forearm, affecting the medial border of the arm and hand.
  - Lower fibers (abdominal division):

    - Referred pain: May cause breast discomfort and nipple hypersensitivity, especially in women. Pressure on the nipple or rubbing against clothing may be uncomfortable.
    - Relation with arrhythmias: A PGM related to somatovisceral cardiac arrhythmias has been described, located in the intercostal space between the fifth and sixth ribs.
  - Parasternal insertional PGMs:
    - Local pain: often referred to the sternum without crossing the midline.
- Clinical implications: The pectoralis major PGMs may shorten, contributing to activation of PGMs in the interscapular musculature (rhomboids and middle trapezius), which may cause pain in this region. There is an association between PGMs of the pectoralis major and superior cruciate syndrome, as well as cervicogenic headaches. Activation of the PGMs may be related to shortening of the muscle, which can generate tension and make postural correction difficult. Activities that involve excessive use of the pectoralis major, such as manual labor and sports that require intense shoulder movement, may be direct mechanisms of activation (57, 58).
- Precordial pain: Precordial pain and armward irradiation of MMPs in the pectoral muscles can be confused with anginal pain, especially if the pain is constant and accompanied by a feeling of constriction in the thorax. This highlights the importance of an accurate diagnosis, as activation of these PGMs could contribute to the persistence of pain after an episode of acute myocardial infarction (57, 58).
- Postoperative considerations: PGMs of the pectoralis major may also be implicated in postoperative pain after mastectomy, causing discomfort in the use of bras and chafing from clothing. The authors have found that these PGMs are frequently involved in frozen shoulder, where they can cause pain and alterations in mobility (57, 58).
- Clinical (57, 58):

- Symptoms: Shortening and biomechanical alterations; intermittent or persistent pain in the anterior aspect of the shoulder, thorax, internal aspect of the upper limb, and breast and nipple hypersensitivity.
- PGM activation: May occur from maintaining a forward shoulder posture, muscle weakness or immobilization.

- PS (57, 58):
  - Technique:
    - Patient position: The patient should be placed in the supine decubitus position.
    - PGM localization: The patient is asked to perform abduction in the plane of the scapula at 90° to make the pectoralis major visible. The central PGMs are located by pincer palpation.
    - Palpation: To facilitate palpation, the patient can be asked to place the hand of the side to be treated on the abdomen, slightly separating the humerus.
    - Puncture: Once the PGM is located, the needle is directed into the clamp towards it, with the usual precautions to avoid accidental puncture of the lung. A 50 mm needle is used in most procedures.
  - Clavicular PGM: For the puncture of the PGMs of the clavicular portion, the physical therapist should locate the tense band using flat palpation. The puncture is performed with a 0.25 mm x 25 mm needle, directing it towards the PGM in a cranial and lateral direction.

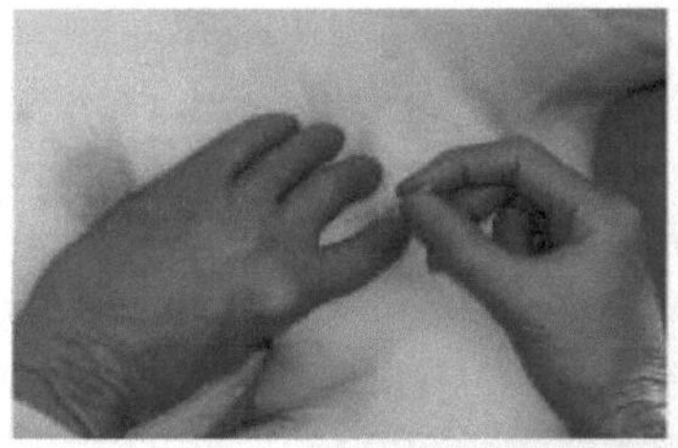

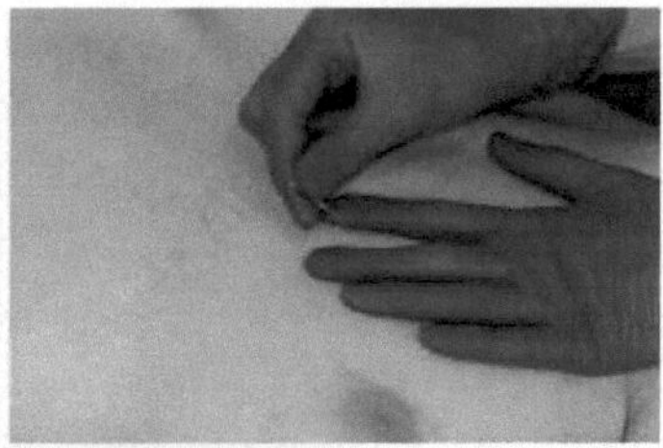

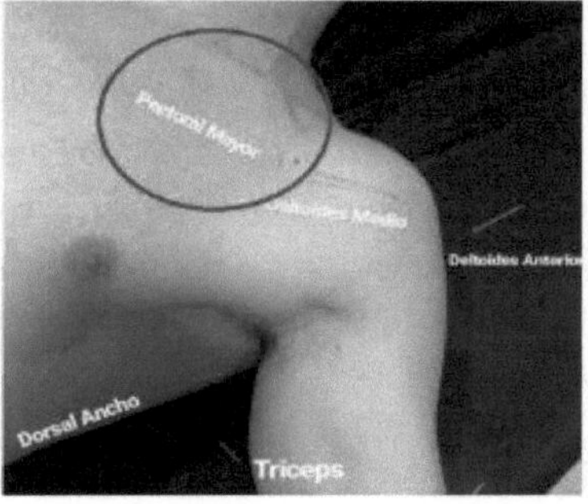

PS in PGM for pectoralis majorale with flat palpation (53, 54).

- Hazards and precautions (57, 58):
  - Pneumothorax: The main complication to avoid is pneumothorax. It is crucial to be attentive to the anatomy and technique to prevent lung puncture.
  - Precautions in patients with breast prostheses: Special care should be taken in patients with breast prostheses, avoiding puncture in nearby areas if the location of the implant cannot be clearly identified.

5.1.5. Pectoralis minor.

- Trigger points and referred pain: The pectoralis minor is a muscle that can generate referred pain mainly in the anterior aspect of the shoulder. However, it can also cause discomfort throughout the homolateral pectoral region and extend down the inner side of the arm to the fingers, especially the latter. Pain originating in the pectoralis minor may mimic cardiac pain, known as pseudoangina pectoris. Because of this possible confusion, it is critical to rule out visceral causes, such as actual angina pectoris or other visceral pathologies, before proceeding with treatments targeting myofascial trigger points (MTrPs) of the pectoral musculature. Shortening of the pectoralis minor, common in the presence of trigger points, can alter the position and motion of the scapula. Increased tension in this muscle can tilt the scapula forward and rotate it downward, affecting arm elevation movements and contributing to problems such as subacromial impaction syndrome. This shortening can also impact the brachial plexus, causing neurological or vascular symptoms, especially during sustained arm elevation. This is known as thoracic gorge syndrome, where the pectoralis minor can compress the neurovascular bundle, generating pain and symptoms related to nerve and vascular entrapment (59, 60).

- PGMs of the pectoralis minor can be activated by a variety of causes, including (59, 60):
  - Prolonged shortening due to bad posture.
  - Direct trauma, overuse in pushing activities, or prolonged use of crutches.
  - Direct compression, such as that caused by the strap of a backpack.
  - Related muscles that can indirectly activate the PGMs of the pectoralis minor include the scalenes, pectoralis major, lower trapezius, and cardiac muscle (viscerosomatic relationship).
- PS technique: The patient should be placed in the supine position, with the homolateral hand on the abdomen to relax the pectoralis major and facilitate palpation of the pectoralis minor. The safest technique for puncture is by clamping the muscle, avoiding the risk of damaging the lung or underlying neurovascular structures (59, 60).

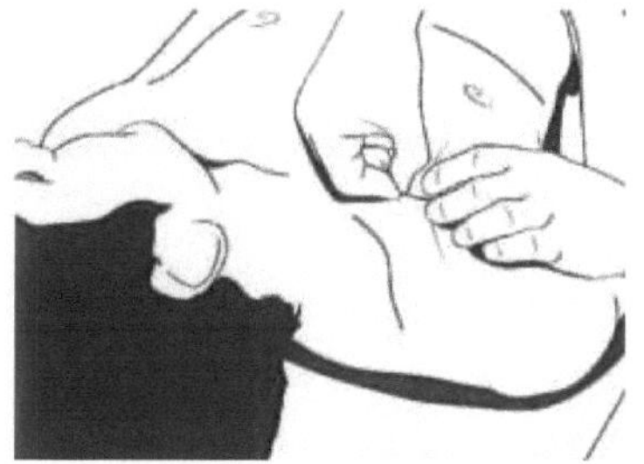
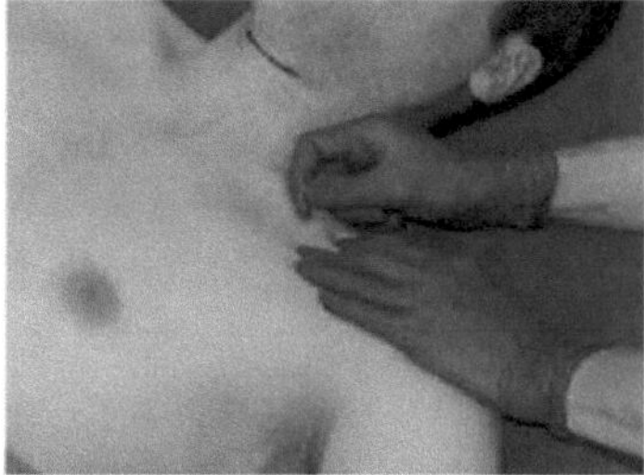

PS in PGM for pectoralis minor with forceps palpation (53, 54).

- Hazards and precautions: The greatest risk of dry needling the pectoralis minor is the development of a pneumothorax if the needle penetrates the lung. There is also the possibility of injuring the brachial plexus or axillary vessels, so it is crucial to perform the puncture with care and adequate hemostasis to avoid bleeding. It is essential to avoid puncture in patients with breast prostheses if the position of the implant cannot be clearly delimited (59, 60).

5.1.6. Subclavian.

- Trigger points and referred pain: The subclavian muscle is a small muscle located under the clavicle, which can present myofascial trigger points (MTrPs) along its entire length, although the most common location is on the lateral part of the medial third of the clavicle. Pain referred by subclavian MTPs may be felt below the clavicle and on the anterior aspect of the arm, radiating to the radial side of the forearm and hand, and even on the anterior aspect of the shoulder. This muscle may contribute to thoracic gorge syndrome, as increased tension or thickening of the subclavian may reduce the costoclavicular space, causing neurovascular compression affecting both the subclavian vessels and the brachial plexus. This can generate neurological and vascular symptoms in the arm (59, 60, 61).
- Clinical (59, 60, 61):
  - Local pain below the clavicle.

- Pain radiating to the anterior aspect of the arm, radial border of the forearm and hand.
- Possible neurological or vascular symptoms due to compression of the subclavian vessels and brachial plexus.

- Related muscles: Scalenes and pectorals (59, 60, 61).
- PS technique: The patient is placed in the supine position, while the therapist is in a cranial position. Deep palpation is performed below the clavicle to locate a tender point, usually in the medial third of the muscle. The puncture should be performed with a 0.25 mm x 25 mm needle, inserting it under the clavicle in a cranial direction until it contacts the bone. The needle is then withdrawn slightly and reoriented to pass through the subclavian space between the clavicle and the ribs. To increase this space and move the muscle away from the thorax, a wedge or folded towel can be placed under the shoulder, which also reduces the risk of pneumothorax (59, 60, 61).

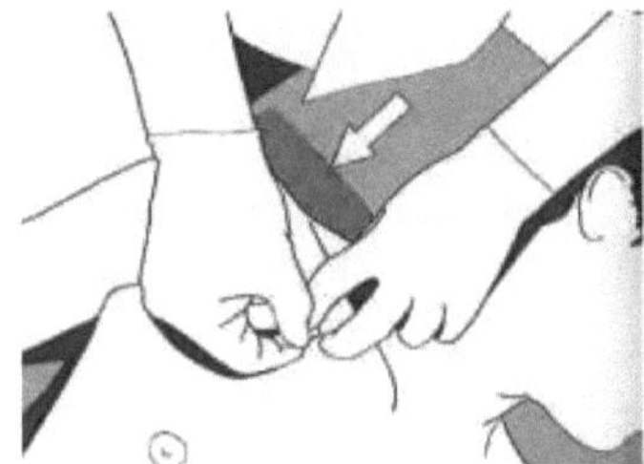
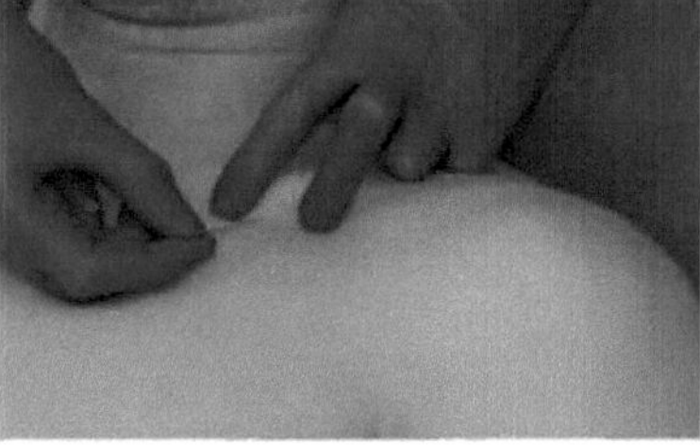

Figure 6. PS in PGM for subclavian (53, 54).

- Dangers and precautions: Because of the proximity to the brachial plexus, subclavian artery and vein, it is important to perform the first needle insertions with caution. The patient should describe whether he/she feels an electrical sensation, which would indicate contact with a nerve, or the characteristic pain of having reached the PGM. After puncture, the area should be compressed to avoid bleeding if a blood vessel has been touched. It is essential to follow the clavicle line to minimize the risk of pneumothorax and to pay special attention to possible vascular effects, given the proximity of large vessels (59, 60, 61).

5.1.7. Thoracic longissimus.

- Trigger points and referred pain: The thoracic longissimus muscle can present myofascial trigger points (MTrPs) along its entire length, from the lowest lumbar fibers to the highest part of the thorax, where they overlap with the fibers of the cervical longissimus and head longissimus. Referred pain symptoms usually follow a line parallel to the spine, descending caudally from the PGM, sometimes radiating to the buttock in the lower thoracic levels, being a frequent cause of lumbar or gluteal pain (62, 63).
- Symptoms and functional limitations: Pain in the trigger points of the longissimus thoracis can limit movements such as rotating the trunk (towards the affected side due to pain and towards the opposite side due to tightness), or hinder forward bending. It also manifests itself in postures that require continuous work of this muscle, such as holding a load with the arms extended away from the body. Examples of these activities include mopping the floor or manual work on a low table, where precision is needed and the weight cannot be aligned with the body. Improper posture or prolonged use of postures such as sitting cross-legged, or in low seating, increase stress on the spinal extensors. These postures can activate or perpetuate PGMs, especially when there is retraction of the pelvitrochanteric or hamstring muscles. In addition, repetitive or sudden activities with trunk flexion, along with trauma or traffic accidents, can trigger bilateral activation of these trigger points. Other causes include body asymmetries, such as leg dysmetry, or habits such as sitting with the wallet in the back pocket. These factors cause imbalances that overload the erector spinae muscles, aggravated by obesity or pregnancy, which generate greater anterior load (62, 63).
- Clinical (62, 63):
  - Lumbar pain radiating to the buttock.
  - Chest pain associated with postural discomfort.

- Limitation of trunk movements.

- Related muscles: Thoracic and lumbar paravertebral muscles. Pelvitrochanteric, iliopsoas, hamstrings (62, 63).
- PS technique: With the patient in prone position, the physical therapist is positioned on the side opposite to the side to be treated. Palpation is performed lateral to the spinous processes, looking for the depression between these and the muscle mass formed by the longissimus and iliocostalis. The first palpable fibers are those of the spinous muscle, although those of the longissimus thoracis are usually easier to identify, since they form a thick cord. The PGMs are located by superficial palpation transverse to the fibers, looking for a taut band with increased tension. Once the PGM is identified, the needle is inserted medially or medially and slightly anteriorly. The size of the needle varies according to the conformation of the patient and the level of the spine. A 0.25 mm x 25 mm needle is commonly used, although a 0.30 mm x 40 mm needle may be necessary in large patients. In some cases, a lateral decubitus approach may be used, adding flexion to the spine to facilitate identification of tight bands and observation of local spasm responses (62, 63).

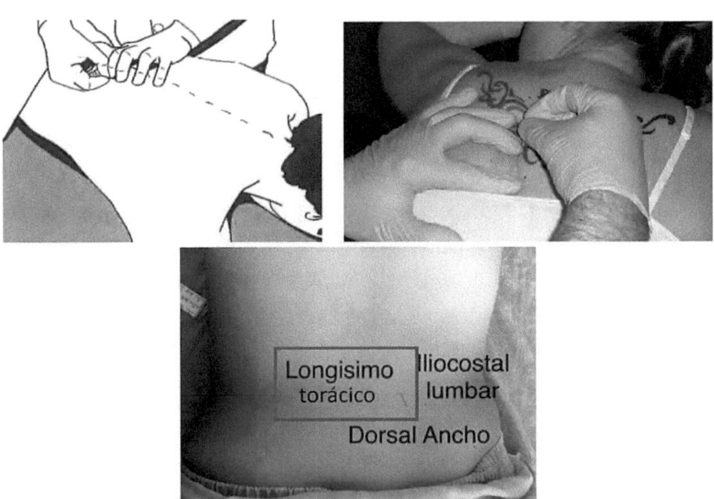

Figure 7. PS in PGM of the thoracic longissimus (53, 54).

- Dangers and precautions: Avoided by inserting the needle in a medial direction, so as not to reach the lung. In patients with pronounced scoliosis, it is necessary to adjust the anatomical references due to the rotation of the spine and ribs, to avoid complications (62, 63).

5.1.8. Thoracic iliocostal.

- Trigger points: The iliocostal muscle, like the thoracic longissimus, is composed of multiple muscle fascicles, which allows finding myofascial trigger points (MTrPs) along the entire muscle, from the lumbar portion to the upper thorax. The MTrPs of this muscle can be located in the lumbar, thoracic or cervical iliocostal (64, 65).
- Referred pain: Referred iliocostal pain may manifest as a line radiating upward, downward, or in a lateral and anterior direction. In the upper and middle thoracic regions, the pain may be confused with visceral problems such as cardiac or pulmonary disease, while in the lower thoracic region it may mimic abdominal pain. This pain may occur in two simultaneous areas: one in the dorsolateral region of the back and the other in the anterolateral region of the thorax. Referred iliocostal PGM pain may also limit spinal movements, either by pain on contraction or by tightness on stretching. In addition, pain may occur with deep breathing (inspiration or expiration), due to the role of this muscle in stabilizing the spine (64, 65).
- Common symptoms (64, 65):
  - Pain next to the spine, radiating cranially, caudally or towards the anterior part of the thorax and abdomen.
  - Limitation of trunk movements, especially bending or rotation.
  - Postural pain or pain related to specific movements.
  - May simulate visceral pathology (cardiac, pulmonary or abdominal).
- Activation mechanisms: The iliocostal may be activated by situations that overload the paravertebral muscles or incorrect

postures. Factors such as: Maintained or incorrect postures (sitting with legs crossed, in very low chairs, etc.). Repetitive or sudden movements of the trunk, especially in flexion or rotation. Trauma, such as traffic accidents, which generate acceleration and deceleration forces. Gravity line imbalances (walking with lower limb problems, scoliosis). Weakness of the deep musculature of the spine, obesity and pregnancy (64, 65).

- Related muscles: Thoracic and lumbar paravertebral muscles. Pelvitrochanteric, iliopsoas and hamstrings. Anterior serratus and external oblique of the abdomen (64, 65).
- Dry needling technique: With the patient in prone position, the physical therapist is positioned on the side opposite the side to be treated. The PGM is located by palpation in the depression lateral to the spinous processes, between the muscle mass of the longissimus and iliocostalis, differentiating both by the texture of the muscle. Once the PGM is located, proceed to puncture with a 0.25 mm x 25 mm needle in the area lateral to the tense band, introducing it in a medial direction, tangential to the thorax (Figure 17-22). In cases where the tense bands are not clearly palpated, the lateral decubitus position with flexion of the spine can be used, which facilitates the identification of the affected muscle (64, 65).

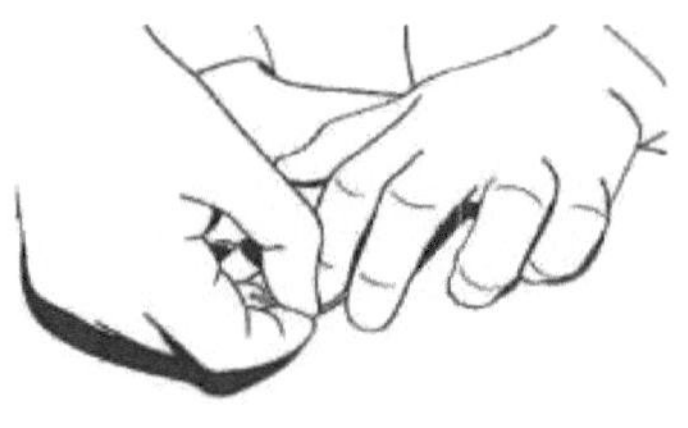

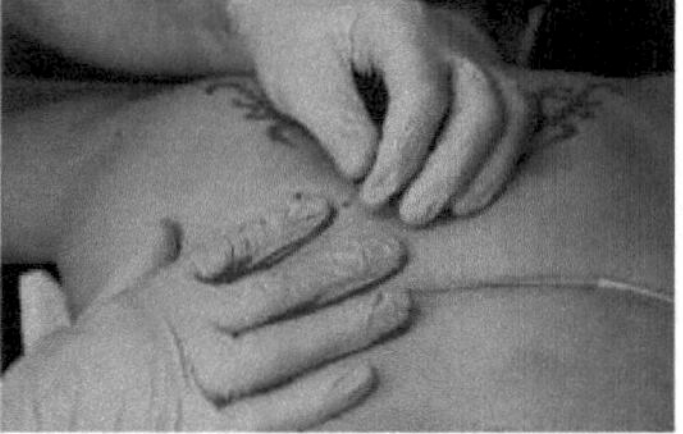

Figure 8. BP in PGM of the thoracic iliocostal (53, 54).

- Hazards and precautions: The greatest risk during puncture is the possibility of causing a pneumothorax if the needle penetrates the lung. This can be avoided by carefully following the medial puncture technique instructions. In patients with scoliosis, anatomical landmarks should be adjusted, as the rotation and arrangement of the ribs and spine may vary (64, 65).

5.1.9. Thoracic multifidus.

- Myofascial trigger points (MTrPs) in the deep paravertebral musculature, such as the transverse spinous muscles, can be found in any segment of the thoracic spine. Referred pain from these points is experienced around the spinous process of the affected vertebra, with pain either central or shifted slightly to the affected side. In some cases, the pain may radiate to the anterior chest wall, giving the sensation of going through the lung. This may require a differential diagnosis with other muscles that can produce similar pain, such as the thoracic iliocostal and posterosuperior serratus (66, 67).
- Referred pain: Pain may be localized in the spine and, in some cases, radiate to the anterior thorax, simulating visceral or deep thoracic pain. Deep palpation may reveal tenderness in the multifidus or rotators, which are components of the transverse spinous musculature. In the affected segment, pain may be unilateral or bilateral, and pain on percussion may be noted in the adjacent spinous process, which may help identify the affected muscle (66, 67).
- Common symptoms (66, 67):
    - Localized or radiating segmental pain, with hypersensitivity in the PGM area.
    - Possible muscle atrophy of the multifidus in chronic conditions, especially in the lumbar and thoracic spine.
    - Stiffness or difficulty in moving the affected vertebral segment.
    - Motor and sensory disturbances, which can be amplified by the presence of PGM and worsen joint dysfunctions.
- PGMs in the transverse spinous muscles can be activated by (66, 67):

- Joint dysfunctions: Changes in joint capsules, ligaments or vertebral discs can induce the activation of these trigger points, particularly in rotators and multifidus.
- Muscle overuse: Incorrect maintained postures or repetitive trunk movements can activate the PGMs in this deep musculature.
- Radiculopathies: Irritation of segmental nerve roots may increase sensitivity and activation of PGMs.
- Segmental sensitization: Persistent pain in one vertebral segment can lead to the appearance of trigger points in the deep musculature, which in turn amplify the pain.

- Dry needling technique: The puncture of the PGMs of the transverse spinous muscles is performed with the patient in prone position. Although tight bands are not always evident, it is possible to detect local changes such as increased density of the subcutaneous tissue, difficulty in mobilizing the skin, and the presence of palpable nodules in the affected area. These signs are key to locate the PGMs. For the procedure, once the PGM is located by palpation, the physiotherapist fixes the point with his finger on the taut band. A 0.30 mm x 40 mm needle is inserted on one side of the spinous process (approximately 1.5 cm), with an orientation of 15° medial to avoid the lung and 15° caudal to avoid the spinal canal. The depth of insertion should be carefully controlled. In people of normal build, if the vertebral lamina has not been reached at 35 mm, the needle should not be deepened further (66, 67).

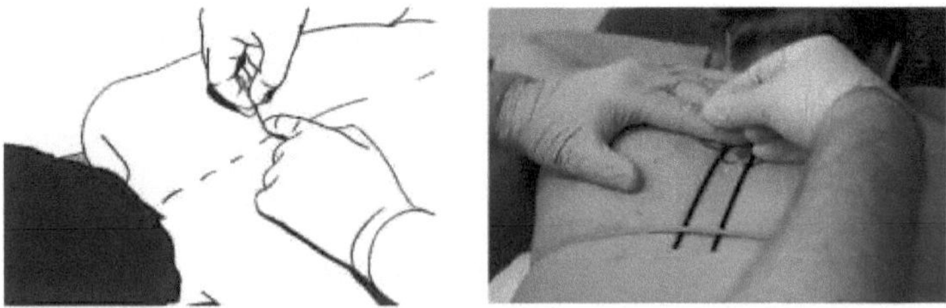

Figure 9. PS for PGM in thoracic multifidus (53, 54).

- Hazards and precautions: There is a risk of pneumothorax if the needle penetrates the lung. To avoid this, it is crucial to follow the medial and caudal orientation of the puncture. In the thoracic region, the risk of entering the spinal canal is low, as long as the needle is correctly oriented. In patients with scoliosis, anatomical landmarks should be adjusted, especially if there is significant spinal rotation. Strict asepsis should be maintained, as the needle could contact the capsule of the zygapophyseal joints during the procedure (66, 67).

5.2. PS for lumbopelvic region.

5.2.1. Lumbar longissimus.

- Myofascial trigger points (MTrPs) in the lumbar longissimus muscle can be found at different levels of the lumbar spine, although they are most common around the L1 vertebra. These points often refer pain toward the posterior iliac crest and sacroiliac joint. They may also radiate to the subgluteal area (near the ischial tuberosity) and, in some cases, to the lumbar region, making this muscle a common contributor to low back pain. The pattern of pain may surprise the patient, as the PGM is often located far from the area that generates the pain. This pattern is responsible for acute low back pain, which significantly limits spinal mobility. In addition, it is associated with other nearby muscles such as the gluteus, piriformis, and hamstrings, which can also develop PGM due to the proximity of the referred pain areas (68).

- Common symptoms (68):
    - Difficulty rising from a sitting or recumbent position and climbing stairs.
    - Reduced spinal mobility, especially when attempting to flex the trunk forward.
    - Acute low back pain that may involve radiating pain to the sacroiliac and subgluteal area.

- Bilateral involvement, which can significantly limit spinal movements.

- The PGMs of the lumbar longissimus can be activated for several reasons (68):
    - Abrupt overload: Rapid or uncontrolled movements of the lumbar spine, such as those occurring in automobile accidents or combined flexion and rotation movements.
    - Chronic overload: Repeated or sustained movements that overload the muscle, such as sitting for prolonged periods of time in bad posture.
    - Axial or pelvic asymmetries: leg length differences, plantar support dysfunctions, or scoliosis can predispose and perpetuate PGMs in this muscle.
    - Joint dysfunctions in the thoracolumbar region: Alterations in the vertebral joints may be an indirect cause of PGM activation.
- Dry needling technique: With the patient in prone or lateral decubitus, a groove containing the tendons of insertion of the lumbar longissimus is palpated lateral to the spinous processes. Because the lumbar longissimus is covered by the lumbar iliocostalis, latissimus dorsi and thoracolumbar fascia, direct palpation is difficult. In the upper lumbar levels, where the iliocostalis is more lateral, it is possible to better identify the location of the longississimus. For this procedure, with the patient in lateral decubitus on the healthy side, the lateral border of the lumbar iliocostalis is located. A transverse puncture is made in a lateromedial direction towards the lumbar longissimus and its MTP. A 0.30 mm x 50 mm needle is used. The puncture can also be performed with the patient in prone position (68).

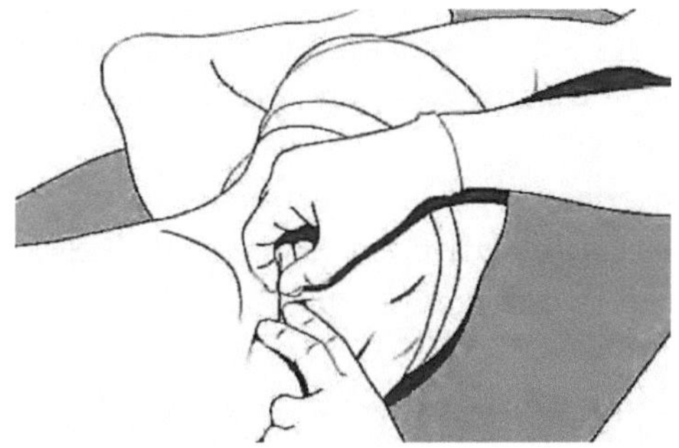

PS in PGM of the lumbar longissimus (53).

- Dangers and precautions: In front of the lumbar longissimus is the quadratus lumborum, and depending on the level treated, the kidney may be encountered. To avoid complications, avoid directing the needle towards the anterior part of the body (68).

5.2.2. lumbar iliocostal.

- Referred pain: Myofascial trigger points (MTrPs) in the lumbar iliocostal muscle can be located at any segmental level, usually within the patient's painful area. This pain radiates caudally, towards the buttock (near the piriformis muscle and gluteus maximus), and may cover the sacroiliac joint. In some cases, the pain radiates cranially or towards the lower costal border and may even affect the hypogastrium or the inguinal region on the same side. When the pain affects the hypogastrium, it may be perceived as a deep visceral pain, which may lead the patient to interpret the discomfort as an abdominal problem (68, 69).
- Common symptoms (68, 69):
  - Pain when getting up, climbing stairs or bending forward, both sitting and standing.
  - Pain on deep breathing or coughing, due to iliocostal involvement in thoracic stabilization.
  - Pain radiating towards the buttock and sacroiliac area, with possible expansion towards the hypogastrium.
- Activation mechanisms (68, 69):

- The lumbar iliocostalis muscle shares the same mechanisms of activation and perpetuation as the lumbar longissimus. These factors include:
- Muscle overload in the lower extremities.
- Pelvic or axial asymmetry: Inequality in the pelvis or spine.
- Biomechanical alterations in plantar support, affecting posture and gait.
- Rapid or uncontrolled movements involving flexion and rotation of the lumbar spine, as in whiplash or traffic accidents.
- Exposure to cold or muscle fatigue.
- In the authors' experience, PGMs in this muscle can also be activated by herpes zoster infections.

- Dry needling technique: The patient is placed in lateral decubitus on the healthy side or in prone position. The PGM and the lateral border of the lumbar iliocostalis muscle are located, which is clearly palpated by moving the tissues from medial to lateral, just behind the quadratus lumborum muscle. The puncture is performed with a 0.30 mm x 50 mm needle, similar to the technique used for the lumbar longissimus muscle (68, 69).

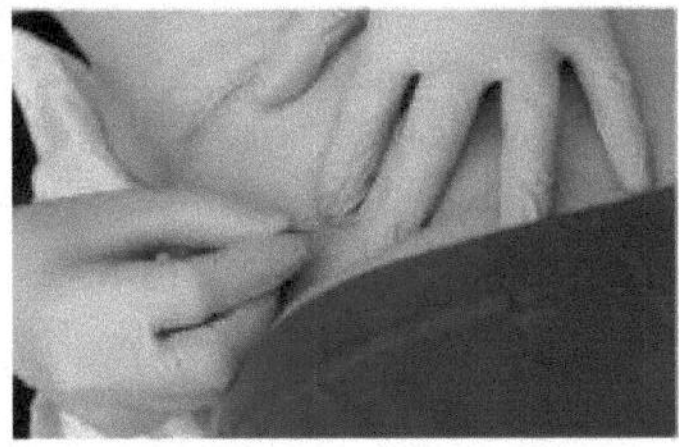

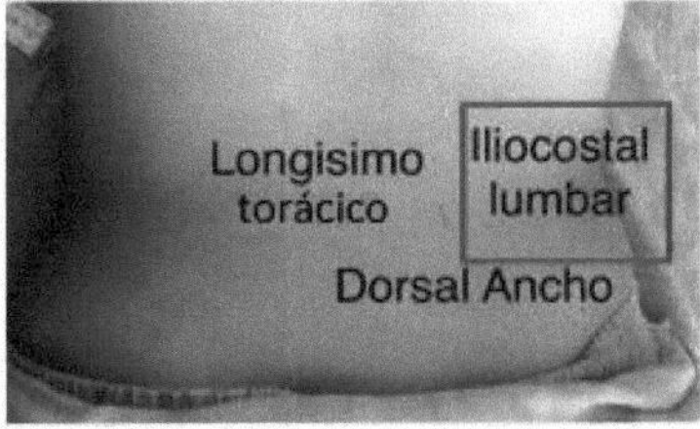

Figure 11. BP in PGM of the lumbar iliocostalis (53).

- Hazards and precautions: The risks and precautions for puncture in the lumbar iliocostal muscle are the same as for the lumbar portion of the lumbar longissimus lumborum, which include the proximity of sensitive structures such as the kidneys, requiring avoidance of the anterior direction of the needle (68, 69).

5.2.3. Lumbar transverse spine.

- Myofascial trigger points (MTrPs) in the lumbar transverse spinal muscles (mainly the multifidus) are difficult to identify due to the absence of tight bands. The referred pain of these PGMs is usually deep and localized around the point itself, with occasional irradiation to the abdomen and areas such as the gluteal area and the anterior and posterolateral aspects of the thigh in cases of low lumbar involvement. This may mimic a lumbar or sacroiliac facet syndrome, and even simulate visceral pain, especially in the abdomen (68, 69, 70).
- Common symptoms (68, 69, 70):
  - Deep and continuous pain, which patients describe as being of bony origin.
  - Pain around the spinous processes, often accompanied by cutaneous hyperalgesia in the overlying skin.
  - Pain on coughing or exertion.
  - Sensation of blockage or restriction in segmental lumbar mobility.
  - In low lumbar PGMs, referred pain may include the thigh and buttocks.
- PGMs in multifids can be activated by several factors (68, 69, 70):
  - Sedentariness and prolonged postures, such as sitting for long periods of time, in flights or administrative jobs.
  - Sudden movements such as accelerations and decelerations in accidents, which stretch the rigid multifid.
  - Axial asymmetries, which contribute to both the activation and perpetuation of PGMs in this muscle group.
  - Muscle weakness in the deep paravertebral or transverse abdominis muscle, whose contraction is closely related to the multifidus. Atrophy or fatty infiltration in the multifidus, common in cases of chronic low back pain, is also associated with the presence of PGM.
- Clinical (68, 69, 70):
  - Pain around the spinous process, with occasional irradiation to the abdomen.

- Hypersensitive coccyx and persistent pain.
- Bone pain, deep and disabling, which may worsen with movement or exertion.
- Lower lumbar PGMs can cause referred pain to the thigh and buttocks.

- Dry needling technique:
  - Patient position: The patient is placed in prone decubitus.
  - Localization: The PGM is located by palpating near the spinous processes. The puncture is performed with a 0.30 mm x 50 mm needle (or 0.30 mm x 60 mm if necessary due to the patient's constitution).
  - Needle insertion: The needle is inserted posteroanteriorly with a caudal inclination of 10°-15°, avoiding penetration of more than 4.5 cm in people of normal constitution to avoid touching the dura mater.

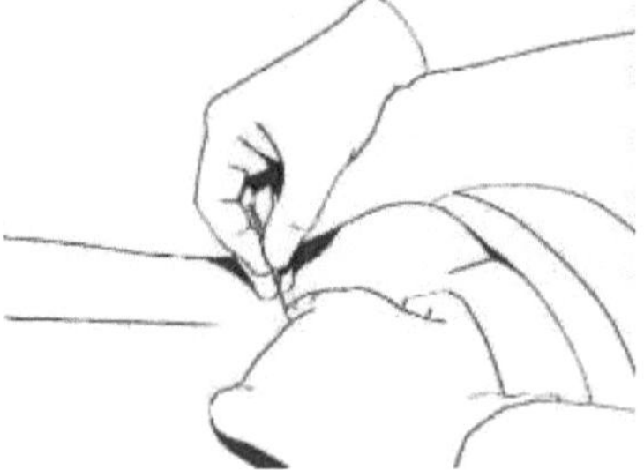

Figure 12. PS in PGM of the lumbar transverse spine (53).

- Hazards and precautions: There is a risk of contacting the dura or penetrating the spinal canal. This is prevented by following proper technique. Caution should be taken when inserting the needle to avoid touching the lumbar zygapophyseal joints, so extreme asepsis measures are recommended. The puncture is contraindicated in cases of spondylolisthesis or spondylolysis, since the relaxation of the deep muscles in these patients could increase vertebral instability (68, 69, 70).

5.2.4. Square lumbar.

- Referred pain: The quadratus lumborum muscle presents myofascial trigger points (MTrPs) in four main areas, which project characteristic pain patterns according to their location (69, 70, 71):
  - Zone 1 (Lateral and cranial): Referred pain in the region just below the iliac crest and may extend to the lower quadrant of the abdomen, groin and sacroiliac joint (SIJ).
  - Zone 2 (Lateral and caudal): The pain is referred to the greater trochanter area and the upper lateral aspect of the thigh.
  - Zone 3 (Medial and cranial): Pain towards the ISA area and, if bilateral, also towards the upper sacral region.
  - Zone 4 (Medial and caudal): The pain projects towards the lower part of the buttock. Occasionally, it may generate a sudden pain that runs down the anterior aspect of the thigh to the knee.

  In addition, some trigger points in the quadratus lumborum are related to referred pain in the genital area (testicles and scrotum) due to the activation of satellite trigger points in the external oblique muscle of the abdomen.
- Common symptoms: Patients usually experience deep, continuous pain at rest, which becomes very sharp and intense with movement, coughing or sneezing. Pain may limit trunk flexion and hinder contralateral rotation and tilt (69, 70, 71).
- Other symptoms include: Need to use arms to get up from a chair, difficulty climbing stairs, disabling pain that may restrict movement, causing the patient to only be able to move around on all fours. Pronounced antalgic position, which the patient may not notice. Referred pain may radiate to the gluteal region, greater trochanter, and is often associated with trigger points in the gluteus minimus, sometimes resulting in pseudociatica (69, 70, 71).
- Activation mechanisms (69, 70, 71):
  - Rapid or repetitive movements, such as lifting weights from a push-up or tilt, can activate the lumbar quadratus PGMs.
  - Traffic accidents and sudden lateral movements are also common triggers.

- Discrepancies in the length of the lower extremities predispose to the activation and perpetuation of these trigger points.

- Related muscles: The quadratus lumborum works in conjunction with muscles such as the gluteus medius, gluteus minimus, iliopsoas, thoracic and lumbar iliocostalis, external oblique and latissimus dorsi (69, 70, 71).
- Dry needling technique (69, 70, 71):
  - Position: The patient is placed in lateral decubitus.
  - The space between the iliac crest and the twelfth rib is identified. The upper leg may be allowed to fall behind the lower leg to facilitate access.
  - The needle is introduced perpendicular to the muscle fibers, with the needle length varying according to the size of the patient (e.g. 0.30 mm x 50 mm for normal persons).

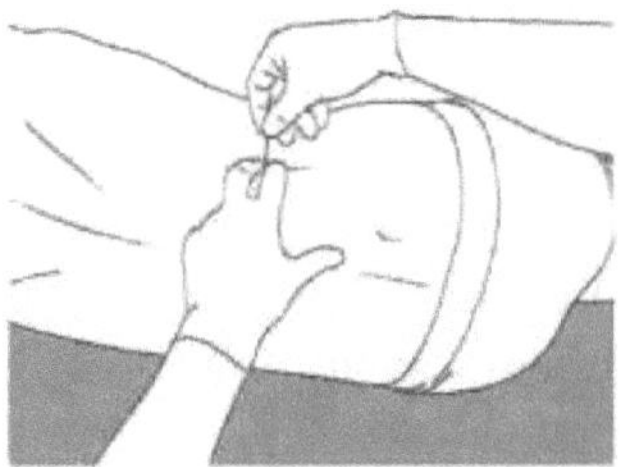
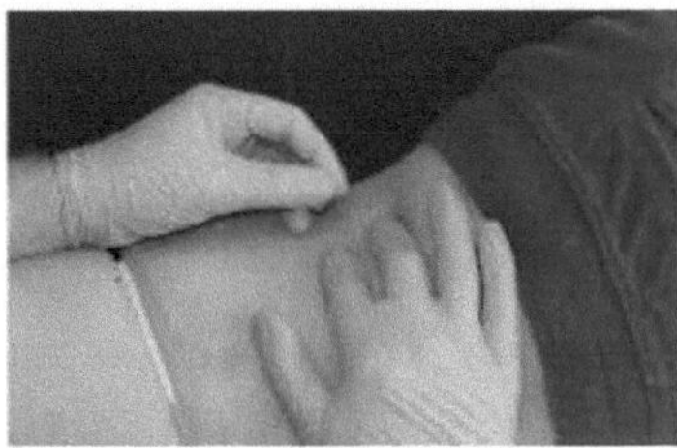

Figure 13. PS in PGM of the lumbar square (53, 54).

- Precautions and hazards: It is important to avoid puncturing the kidney, especially in thin people, making sure that the needle remains in the safe plane of the back (69, 70, 71).
- Other risks include: Puncture of the lung by inserting the needle incorrectly in the upper area and irritation of the iliohypogastric and ilioinguinal nerves, which can cause painful sensations in the innervated areas (gluteal region, thigh, scrotum, penis, etc.) (69, 70, 71).

5.2.5. Iliopsoas.

- PGMs can be located in both the psoas major and the iliacus, especially in the tendon area in the inguinal region. In the latter location, the psoas major is mainly tendinous, so PGMs in this area are more attributed to the iliacus muscle (72, 73).
- Referred iliopsoas pain usually projects vertically along the lumbar paravertebral region, extending to the sacroiliac joint (SIJ) and the proximal and medial buttock. It may also include the inguinal region and the anterosuperior aspect of the thigh, the latter pattern being more characteristic of inguinal PGMs. It has been observed that iliopsoas pain can radiate to the knee, genitalia (scrotum or labia) or even to the interscapular region. Occasionally, psoas minor PGMs can cause homolateral abdominal pain, similar to appendicitis when it occurs on the right side (72, 73).
- Symptoms and behavior of the pain: When the involvement is unilateral, patients usually point out the location of the pain by moving the hand vertically over the affected lumbar area. In case it is bilateral, this verticality is lost, showing the pain transversely, as if it were referred pain of the lumbar quadratus lumborum. It is not uncommon for the PGMs of both muscles to be activated concomitantly. Patients are usually worse when standing and find relief when lying on their side or sitting with knees and hips flexed. They often experience pain in the anterosuperior thigh, especially during contraction into hip flexion. Many report difficulty sitting up from the supine position or from a low chair, accompanied by a feeling of stiffness on hip extension. In addition, iliopsoas PGMs can cause muscle weakness and pain on trunk extension (72, 73).
- Clinical evaluation in patients with acetabular syndromes, labral lesions or hip prostheses, it is advisable to evaluate the presence of MMP in the iliopsoas (72, 73).
- Clinical symptoms (72, 73):
    - Vertical lumbar pain in unilateral or transverse involvement in bilaterality.
    - Pain on rising from the supine position.
    - Relief in lateral decubitus.

- Pain in the anterosuperior aspect of the thigh.

- Mechanisms of PGM activation: The iliopsoas PGMs can be activated directly by falls or by remaining in a curled-up position for prolonged periods of time (e.g., sitting in a low chair, driving, or sleeping in the fetal position). They can also be perpetuated by improper sit-ups, forced hyperextension of the trunk, and straining, especially when climbing slopes. However, indirect mechanisms appear to be more frequent. These include PGM activation in other muscles such as the iliocostalis, quadratus lumborum, hamstrings, rectus femoris, among others. They may also be related to axial dysmetries, degenerative pathologies of the hip and joint dysfunctions in the lumbosacral region (72, 73).
- Muscles related to the iliopsoas PGMs include: Quadratus lumborum, longissimus thoracis, iliocostalis thoracis and lumbaris, gluteus maximus and medius, tensor fascia latae, pectineus, vastus intermedius, adductors (72, 73).
- PS (72, 73):
  - To locate the psoas major PGMs: The patient is placed in the supine position with the hip in active 90-degree flexion and the abdomen relaxed. The fingers are placed approximately midway along an imaginary line between the anterior superior iliac spine (ASIS) and the umbilicus, applying gentle pressure posteriorly and medially. Deepen slowly until the muscle (a cylindrical mass, slightly oblique downward and outward) is felt. Palpation can be checked by asking the patient to relax the muscle intermittently. When the most sensitive area is located, its level in relation to the iliac crest is noted for future reference in invasive treatment.
  - Approach for puncture: The patient is placed in lateral decubitus on the healthy side, with both hips flexed at 90 degrees. If the PGMs are at L4, the approach is made 4-4.5 cm lateral to the spinous process of L4. The puncture is performed with a 0.30 mm x 75 mm needle, in a posteroanterior direction with a medial tilt of about 45 degrees. For more caudal PGMs,

at the approximate height of L5, a 75 mm long needle is used, except in thin patients, where 60 mm needles are recommended.

- Localization of PGMs in the iliacus: The iliacus PGMs can be located at any height of the muscle, being accessible to palpation below the iliac crest ridge. The physiotherapist palpates the PGM on the internal aspect of the iliacus with the patient in the supine position, hip and knee flexed. The 0.25 mm x 40 mm needle is introduced close to the iliac crest, in a posterior and lateral oblique direction.
- PGMs in the inguinal region: To palpate and treat PGMs in the inguinal region, the patient is placed in the supine position. The sartorius muscle, which forms the lateral border of the femoral triangle, is located. Medial to the sartorius is the iliopsoas. The PGMs in this area may be superficial and palpable, although they are generally deeper, requiring a long needle (0.30 mm x 50 mm) for puncture in the anteroposterior direction, avoiding the medial direction so as not to damage the femoral nerve.

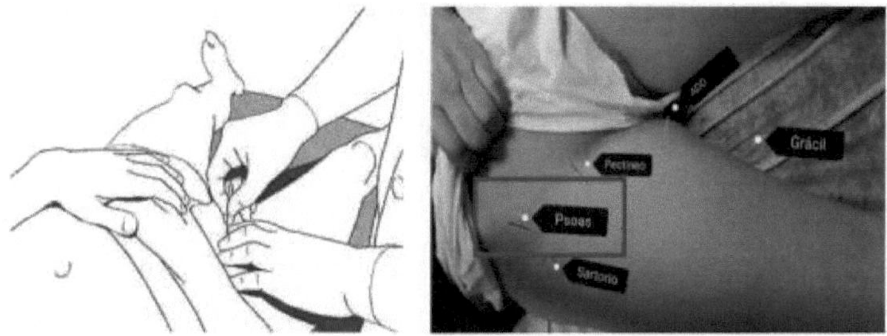

Figure 14. PS in PGM for iliopsoas (53).

- Risks and precautions: Puncture at each iliopsoas PGM location carries risks. It is important to follow precautions to avoid complications (72, 73):
  - Psoas Major: There is a risk of damaging the kidney if the needle is introduced too laterally. The puncture must be performed

under conditions of maximum asepsis, especially in patients with coagulopathies or under treatment with anticoagulants.

- Iliac: Care must be taken with the lateral femoral cutaneous nerves and the branches of the iliohypogastric and ilioinguinal nerves, as well as avoiding penetration into the abdominal cavity.
- Inguinal: It is crucial to take measures to avoid damaging the neurovascular bundle, especially the femoral nerve, which is medial to the muscle in this area.

5.2.6. Gluteus maximus.

- The gluteus maximus muscle is divided into four zones where PGMs can be located (74, 75, 76):
  - Zone 1:
    - Location: Near the lateral/superior border of the gluteus maximus.
    - Referred Pain: Pain in the muscle itself and nearby areas of the buttock.
    - Note: This area may overlap with the gluteus medius and gluteus minimus muscles, complicating the identification of the muscle causing the hyperalgesia.
  - Zone 2:
    - Location: Immediately adjacent to zone 1, overlapping the piriformis muscle.
    - Referred Pain: Pain along the medial aspect of the gluteus maximus, homolateral SIJ, subgluteal fold and proximal thigh.
  - Zone 3:
    - Location: In the subgluteal crease, near the ischial tuberosity.
    - Referred Pain: Pain that extends throughout the buttock, the lower part of the sacrum and below the iliac crest. Pressure at this point can be very painful.
  - Zone 4:

    - Location: In the intergluteal fold.
    - Referred pain: Local pain radiating to the coccyx, may cause coccygodynia.
- PGMs in the gluteus maximus can be activated by (74, 75, 76):
  - Acute eccentric overload (falls or sudden movements).
  - Direct hits.
  - Prolonged uphill walking.
  - Intramuscular injections.
  - In addition, factors such as swimming crawl, carrying in the posterior pocket, having Morton's foot or standing postures with kyphosis can perpetuate PGMs.
- Patients with MGP in the gluteus maximus may present with symptoms such as: persistent pain and discomfort when sitting, limitation in hip flexion, weakness, pain that increases when climbing slopes, especially with anterior flexion or swimming crawl (74, 75, 76).
- Dry puncture (SP): Position of the patient in lateral decubitus on the healthy side (74, 75, 76):
  - Zone 1, 3 and 4: Upper leg behind the lower leg.
  - Zone 2: Hip of the upper leg in front of the lower leg with a flexion of approximately 80º.
  - Puncture techniques:
    - Zone 1: 0.30 mm x 75 mm needle recommended.
    - Zone 2: Overlapping with the piriformis is sought for simultaneous puncture.
    - Zone 3: Use of a 0.30 mm x 50 mm needle, avoiding the sciatic nerve.
    - Zone 4: Clamp palpation, directing the needle towards the finger on the opposite side.

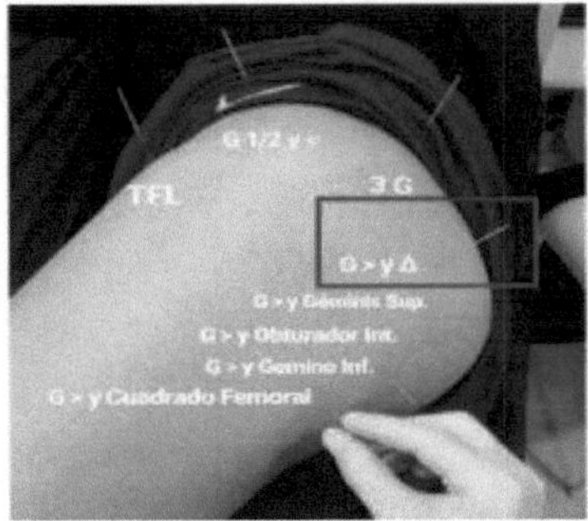

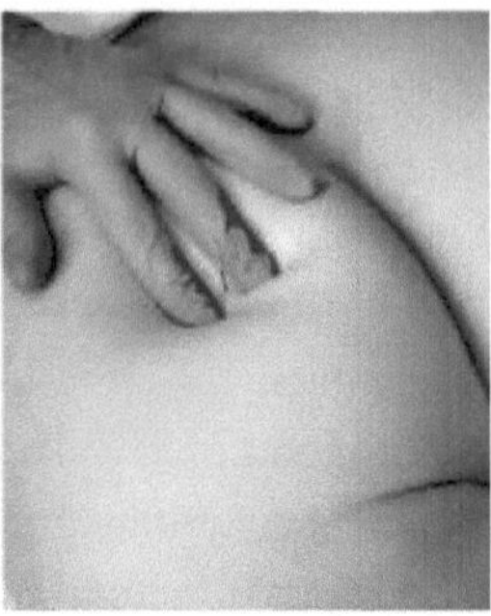

Figure 15. PS in PGM of the gluteus maximus.

- Dangers and precautions: Accidental puncture of the sciatic nerve. The above indications and precautions should be followed to avoid complications (74, 75, 76).

5.2.7. Gluteus medius.

- PGMs of the gluteus medius can be found in different areas of the muscle (74, 75, 76):
  - Central zone: You can have PGMs in any part of the muscle, mainly in the central zone of the fibers.
  - Posterior fibers: Pain extending along the iliac crest, lumbar area, half of the homolateral sacrum, ASI and almost the entire buttock.
  - Medial fibers: Refers to the medial part of the gluteus and the posterior-lateral area of the thigh, including the greater trochanter of the femur.
  - Anterior fibers: May extend along the iliac crest, lower lumbar region and bilaterally over the sacrum.
  - In addition, it has been observed that gluteus medius PGMs can simulate sciatic pain and that they are related to gluteus minimus PGMs, as both share mechanisms of activation and perpetuation.
- PGMs in the gluteus medius can be activated for a variety of reasons (74, 75, 76):

- Direct trauma: Includes injuries from sports or falls.
- Chronic overload: antalgic gait, lower limb dysmetry, pronated foot, sudden changes of direction or running on uneven terrain.
- Interaction with other Muscles: For example, the PGMs of the quadratus lumborum can activate PGMs in the gluteus medius due to their role in the lateral stabilization of the pelvis.

- Patients with MGP in the gluteus medius may experience symptoms such as: pain when walking and in positions that compress the muscle, difficulty sleeping in lateral decubitus on the affected side or in supine decubitus if the MGP are in the most posterior fibers. The referred pain can be confused with ISA dysfunctions, affecting also the gluteus minimus in many cases (74, 75, 76).
- Dry needling: position the patient in lateral decubitus on the healthy side, with the lower leg in hip flexion and the upper leg behind, in slight adduction. If the position is uncomfortable or causes pain, a support can be placed under the knee to limit the stretching of the muscle. For the puncture technique, the superior vertex of the greater trochanter, the iliac crest and the anterior border of the gluteus maximus are used as references. Transverse palpation is performed to the middle part of the fibers. Regarding the needles for the posterior (covered in part by the gluteus maximus) and medial areas of the gluteus medius, a 0.30 mm x 75 mm needle is recommended. For the anterior part, a 0.30 mm x 60 mm needle is suggested (74, 75, 76).

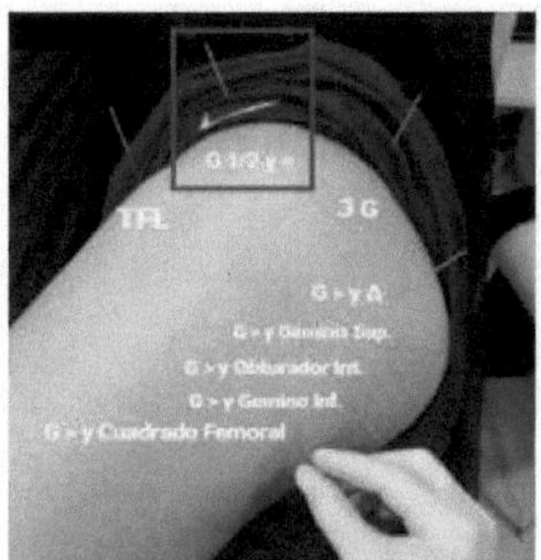

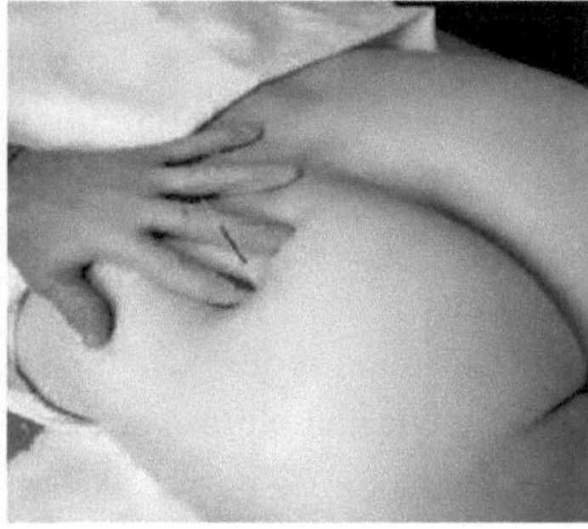

Figure 16. PS in PGM of the gluteus medius (54).

- Dangers and precautions: Branches of the superior gluteal neurovascular bundle pass between the gluteus medius and gluteus minimus, which increases the risk of complications during puncture. Strictly follow the rules for puncture in areas close to nerves, as described in the corresponding chapter (74, 75, 76).

5.2.8. Gluteus minimus.

- The gluteus minimus PGMs are located deep in the gluteal region and their referred pain can be felt in the buttock and throughout much of the lower limb. Pain patterns are divided according to the anterior and posterior portions of the muscle (74, 75, 76):
  - Anterior fibers: referred pain inferolateral to the buttock, outer thigh, knee and peroneal region of the leg, up to the ankle. Rarely, it may reach the dorsum of the foot.
  - Posterior fibers: referred pain inferomedia of the buttock, posterior aspect of the thigh, calf and sometimes the back of the knee.
- PGMs of the gluteus minimus can cause symptoms such as (74, 75, 76):
  - Pseudoradicular syndromes:
    - Anterior fibers: Simulate an L5 radiculopathy.
    - Posterior Fibers: May mimic S1 radiculopathy.
  - Additional symptoms:
    - Intense and persistent pain, which may be constant and sharp.
    - Difficulty walking, limping, and pain that interferes with sleep (especially when in lateral recumbency or sitting).
    - Difficulties to sit up after sitting.
- The gluteus minimus PGMs can be activated by several factors (74, 75, 76):
  - Overload: sudden (falls), repetitive (walking on uneven terrain, antalgic gait, sports activities), chronic (lower limb dysmetria).
  - Other Causes: ISA dysfunctions, intramuscular injections, radicular irritation, prolonged immobility (driving or standing),

pelvic tilt from sitting on a hard surface, interaction with other muscles, such as the quadratus lumborum and other related muscles.

- Dry puncture (74, 75, 76):
  - Puncture Technique: The technique is similar to that of the gluteus medius. A good localization of the PGMs is required to perform the puncture properly.
  - Precautions: Lancing of the gluteus minimus is contraindicated in cases of coagulation disturbances. A transient sensation of weakness and heaviness in the affected limb may occur after the puncture, which may cause lameness for several hours.

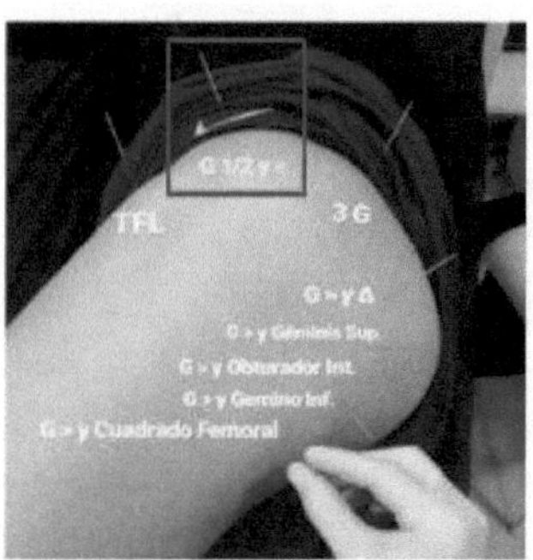

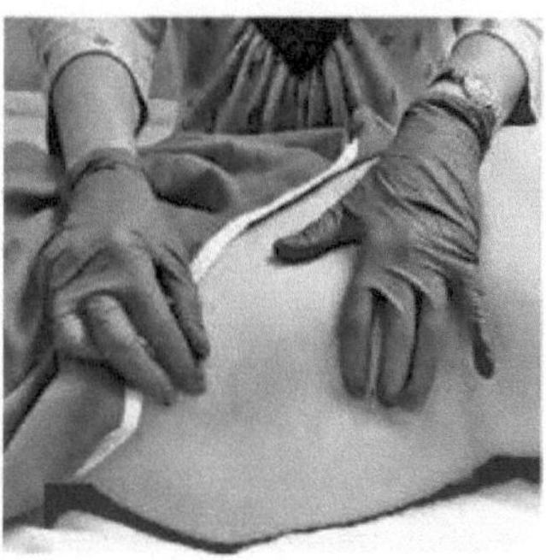

Figure 17. PS in PGM of the gluteus minimus (54).

- Dangers and precautions: The same as those described for the gluteus medius, with the addition that, due to the depth of the muscle, additional caution is necessary. There may be transient muscle inhibition after puncture, manifesting as weakness or heaviness, which is important to communicate to the patient prior to the procedure (74, 75, 76).

5.2.9. Tensor of the fascia lata (TFL).

- TFL PGMs cause referred pain in the hip joint and the anterolateral aspect of the thigh, which may extend to the knee. There are variations in the pattern of referred pain that can be observed (77).

- Referred pain pattern: pain in the greater trochanter, which may be confused with trochanteric bursitis. Some patients report referred pain in the lumbar and sacral area, related to tension in the iliotibial band, especially in runners (77).
- Symptoms: Pain is accentuated during hip movement, especially with rapid walking. Increases with prolonged sitting (especially in 90° hip flexion position). Difficulty sleeping, patients often sleep supine and have difficulty turning laterally on the affected side due to pressure on the muscle and greater trochanter. It may be necessary to place a pillow between the legs to relieve pain (77).
- Differential diagnosis: The diagnosis should consider other PGMs, such as those of the anterior fibers of the gluteus medius and gluteus minimus, vastus lateralis, piriformis and quadratus lumborum (77).
    - Neuropathies: Neuropathies should also be considered, L4 neuropathy and meralgia paresthetica can cause pain in similar areas.
    - Iliotibial Tape Friction Syndrome: Diffuse pain in the lateral condyle of the femur due to friction of the iliotibial tract, especially relevant in runners with pronated feet.
    - Sacroiliitis: It can refer pain to the lumbar and lateral thigh, sometimes reaching the knee.
- TFL PGMs can be activated by a variety of factors (77):
    - Acute overload: From activities such as kicking a ball, running uphill or falls.
    - Chronic overload: Activities such as jogging or walking with hyperpronated feet or on inclined surfaces.
    - Maintenance in a Cramped Position: Sedentation or decubitus with very flexed hips.
    - Dysfunctions: Of the coxofemoral joint or the presence of PGMs in related muscles, such as the quadratus lumborum or adductors.
- Related muscles (77):

- Agonist muscles: gluteus minimus, gluteus medius, sartorius, rectus femoris, iliopsoas.
- Antagonist muscles: hamstrings, gluteus maximus, hip adductors.

- Dry needling (77):
  - Lancing technique: The patient is placed in supine decubitus with the limb stretched. The anterior border of the TFL is located, asking the patient to perform a slight active hip flexion. The taut bands and PGMs are identified in order to proceed with the puncture, directing the needle perpendicularly to the fibers of the taut band.
  - Needle size: For punctures in the TFL the needle is 0.25 mm x 40 mm or 0.30 mm x 60 mm if the anterior part of the gluteus minimus is to be included.

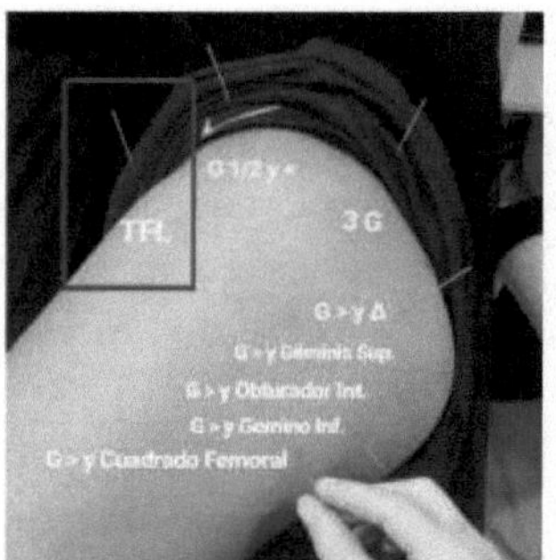

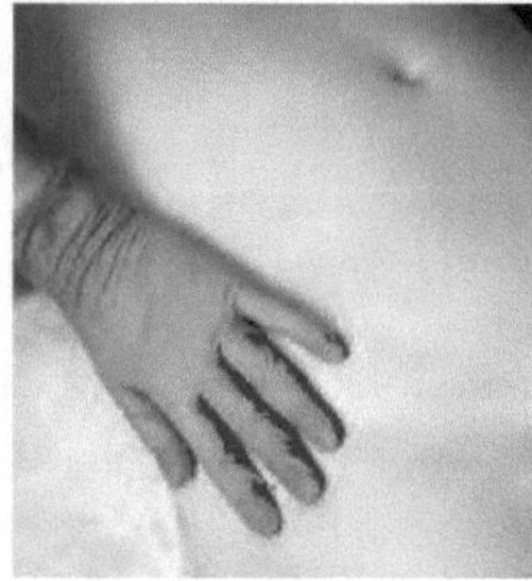

Figure 18. PS in PGM of the TFL (54).

- Dangers and precautions: Although few, care should be taken with cutaneous branches of the superior gluteal nerve passing through the muscle. Follow proper instructions to avoid damaging the nerve (77).

5.2.10. Piriform.

- Location and frequency: The PGMs of the piriformis muscle are commonly located in the lateral half and in the proximal part of the muscle, the lateral ones being easier to identify by palpation (78, 79).

- Referred pain from these points may radiate to: Sacroiliac region, buttocks, posterior hip, posterior thigh (proximal two-thirds). It may also be confused with pain from other hip external rotator muscles (78, 79).
- Associated syndromes: Piriformis PGMs can contribute to several painful syndromes in the pelvis and hip, including piriformis syndrome. It is crucial to make a differential diagnosis with conditions such as disc herniation, lumbosacral radiculopathy, sacroiliitis, and tumor and other pathologies (78, 79).
- Activation mechanisms (78, 79):
  - Direct mechanisms: Trauma, forced eccentric contractions, prolonged positions that shorten the muscle, and compression by neighboring structures.
  - Indirect mechanisms: PGM in paravertebral and gluteal muscles, as well as chronic infections and joint degeneration.
- Clinical features of the syndrome include: Referred pain pattern, weakness on hip abduction, pain on pressure in the muscle, neurological examination is essential to rule out more serious problems (78, 79).
- Treatment: Dry needling is performed with the patient in contralateral decubitus and the hip flexed. The puncture should be guided by EMG or ultrasound to minimize the risk of damage to nerves such as the sciatic. Needle size 0.30 mm x 50 mm. 60 mm or 75 mm (78, 79).

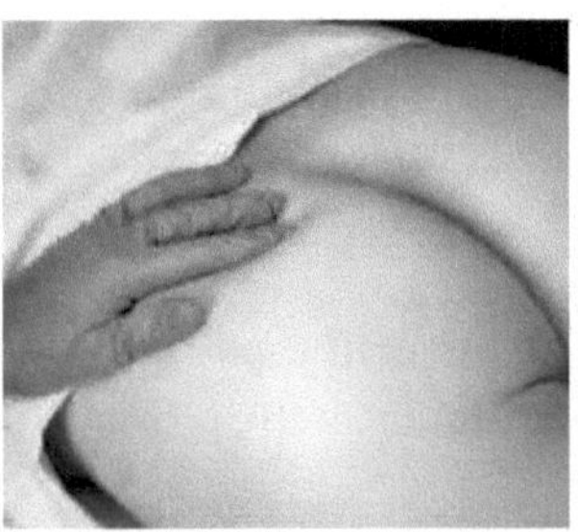 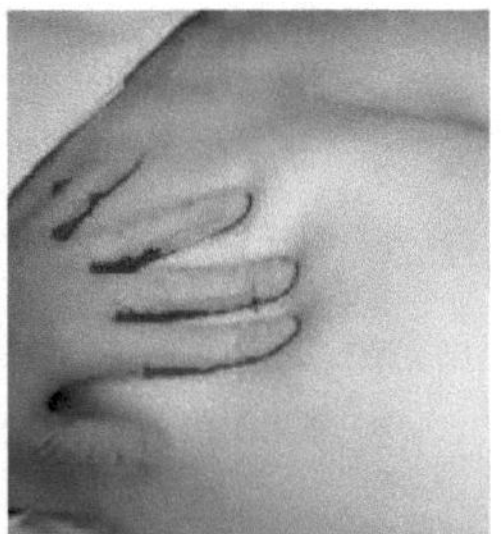

Figure 19. PS in PGM of the piriformis (origin and insertion) (54).

- Risks and precautions: There is a risk of accidental puncture of nerve structures and possibility of entering the pelvis laterally, risk of touching the coxofemoral joint. Asepsis measures must be followed and the depth of the puncture carefully monitored to avoid complications (78, 79).

5.2.11. Rectus abdominis.

- PGMs can be located anywhere in the rectus abdominis muscle. Although symptoms may vary between different areas of the muscle and between individuals, generally, PGMs located in the upper portion of the abdomen (above the umbilicus) tend to cause bilateral posterior horizontal pain, especially in the mid-back. If the pain is unilateral, it is often related to the latissimus dorsi muscle (80,81).
- PGMs can cause pain in the region between the costal ridges and the xiphoid process, causing symptoms similar to those of the transverse abdominis, including abdominal fullness, burning and indigestion. Specifically, if the PGM is on the left side, nausea, vomiting and precordial pain may occur. PGMs in the periumbilical region, located at the lateral border of the muscle, are responsible for diffuse abdominal pain, especially when moving, as well as cramping or colicky sensations, common in children. In the lower part of the muscle, the PGMs located between the umbilicus and the pubic symphysis can cause dysmenorrhea. In the lower rectus abdominis, they may refer bilateral pain to the lumbosacral region, and the patient describes it with a transverse movement of the hand, as opposed to the vertical pain characteristic of the psoas major. A possible PGM area at the superior border of the pubis that may refer pain to the bladder and cause diarrhea. In addition, spasm in this area may result in increased urinary frequency, urinary retention, and groin pain, especially in children. A PGM at the lateral border of the rectus abdominis, near McBurney's point (equidistant from the anterosuperior iliac spine and the umbilicus),

can mimic symptoms of acute appendicitis, causing pain throughout the abdomen, iliac fossa and penis. If the pain is due to appendicitis, global rigidity of the abdominal muscles is present. Given the risk of false positives in the diagnosis of appendicitis, it is reasonable to consider abdominal PGMs in the differential diagnosis (80,81).

- It is crucial to differentiate symptoms of visceral origin from those of muscular origin, since they often coexist. If the pain is muscular, the patient experiences mechanical pain, related to movement and unrelated to food intake or evacuation. Prolonged activities requiring forced abdominal breathing may also exacerbate the pain. Carnett's test may be useful for differential diagnosis. It consists of pressing a painful spot and asking the patient to contract the muscle. If the pain increases, it indicates a muscular origin; if it decreases, it is more likely to be an intra-abdominal problem (80,81).
- PGMs can be caused by mechanical overload, trauma, incorrect posture or indirect factors such as infections, emotional stress and joint dysfunction. Surgical scars, especially after appendicitis, hysterectomies and cesarean sections, can cause myofascial problems in the abdominal and lumbar musculature, perpetuating PGMs (80,81).
- Dry needling, combined with conservative treatment, is often effective in treating the abdominal musculature. Superficial puncture is recommended as a first option, followed by dry needling electrotherapy if necessary. If these techniques do not work, deep dry needling may be considered. The procedure involves identifying tense bands and PGMs while the patient is supine. A 0.25 mm x 40 mm needle is used, inserting it carefully to avoid damaging the peritoneal cavity. The puncture must be performed with rigorous antiseptic measures to prevent infection (80,81).

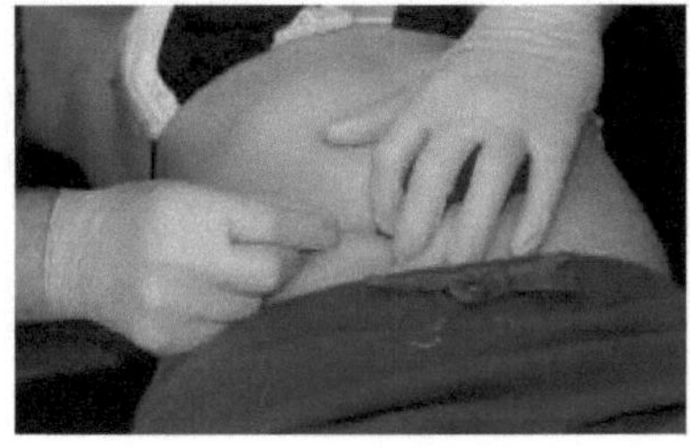 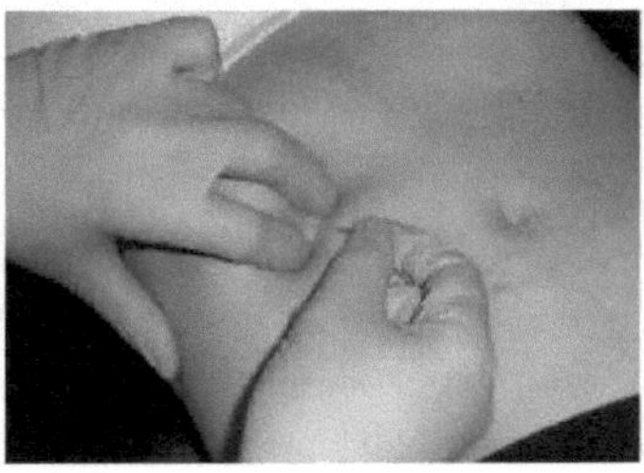

PS in PGM of the rectus abdominis (54).

- Risks: When treating abdominal PGMs, it is vital to evaluate the presence of other factors that may contribute to pain, such as the presence of neurological syndromes that may mimic gynecological conditions in women. Correct identification and treatment of PGMs is essential for patient recovery and improvement of quality of life (80,81).

5.2.12. External oblique of the abdomen.

- PGMs in the abdominal muscles, especially in the external oblique, are areas of tension that can cause symptoms such as heartburn, pain in the epigastrium, and referred pain to the groin and testicles. This can be confused with problems such as hiatal hernia or appendicitis, since the pain can radiate to other areas of the abdomen (82).
- PGMs can be activated by (82):
  - Direct blows: Trauma or impact to the abdominal region.
  - Repetitive Trunk Movements: Activities involving rotation or flexion-extension, such as throwing discs.
  - Maintained positions: Keeping the trunk in rotation may contribute to trigger point activation.
- Referred pain patterns (82):
  - Superior PGMs: Located in the superior part of the external oblique, these can cause burning and epigastric pain.
  - Inferior PGMs: Located in the inferior part, they may refer pain to the groin and testicle, also affecting the opposite side.

- Dry needling: Dry needling is a treatment used to treat PGMs, involving the insertion of needles into the affected muscles to relieve pain. The technique varies according to the location of the PGMs (82):
    - Upper PGMs: Use 0.25 mm x 13 mm needles, inserting them perpendicular to the PGM.
    - Lower PGMs (below EIAS):
        - Palpate the area with the hip in extension to identify tight bands.
        - Use needles of 0.25 mm x 25 mm or 0.25 mm x 40 mm depending on the thickness of the fabric.
    - PGM Over the iliac crest: Palpation in forceps to avoid damaging viscera, with needles of at least 0.25 mm x 40 mm.

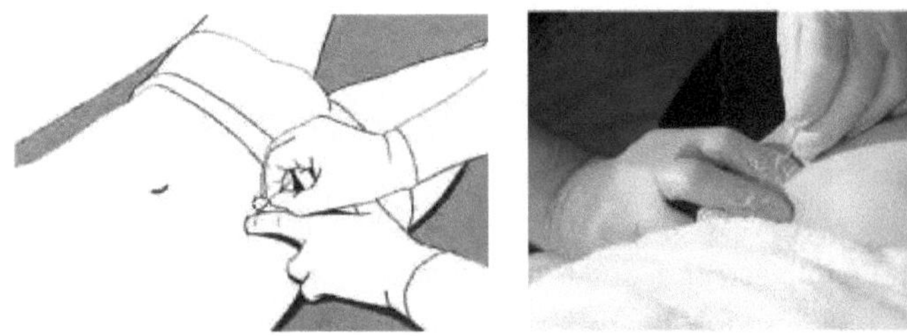

Figure 21. PS in PGM of the external oblique of the abdomen (53, 54).

- Precautions and risks: It is crucial to avoid puncture of the peritoneum, following strict hygiene protocols and proper puncture techniques. The depth of insertion must be carefully evaluated, and ultrasound-guided or EMG-guided puncture is recommended for greater precision and safety (82).

5.2.13. Internal oblique of the abdomen.

- PGM symptoms and activation: Trigger points (PGMs) in the lower and lateral abdominal musculature can cause referred pain to various areas, including the groin, testicle and other areas of the abdomen, and even the chest or opposite side of the abdomen. This pattern of pain can originate from any of the lateral abdominal muscles, such as the obliques and transverse abdominis. The internal oblique and rectus abdominis are particularly responsible for PGMs located at the superior border of the pubis and the lateral half of the inguinal ligament, which can cause urinary bladder pain and muscle spasms related to urination. In addition, the internal oblique and transverse abdominis may be involved in ilioinguinal nerve entrapment, a condition that can arise as a complication of abdominal surgeries or during pregnancy and childbirth, causing significant pain (82, 83).

- PGMs may also be related to other muscles, such as: diaphragm, paravertebral (superficial and deep), serratus anterior, iliopsoas, hip adductors (82, 83).
- Dry puncture: For the treatment of PGMs, a superficial dry puncture (DP) combined with conservative treatment is recommended. It is essential to follow rigorous aseptic measures to avoid infection, especially if there is a risk of penetrating the peritoneal cavity (82, 83).
    - Location of PGMs: The most common location of internal oblique PGMs is medial to the anterior superior iliac spine (ASIS). The puncture technique and the way to determine the depth are similar to those used for the PGMs of the external oblique.
    - Puncture depth: The use of 0.25 mm x 40 mm needles is recommended. According to studies, the puncture depth can be between 13 mm in women and 18 mm in men, minimizing the risk of penetrating the peritoneal cavity.

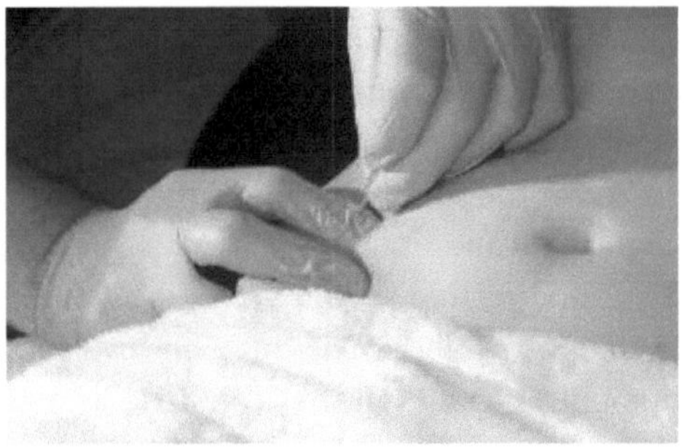

Figure 22. PS in PGM of the internal oblique of the abdomen (54).

- Dangers and precautions: It is vital to avoid inserting the needle into the peritoneum. To this end, the following precautions should be taken (82, 83):
    - Antiseptic measures: Extreme hygiene during the procedure.
    - Follow-up of Protocols: Perform the puncture following the previously described procedures, ensuring correct needle placement and avoiding complications.

5.2.14. Transversus abdominis.

- Symptoms and activation mechanisms: Trigger points (PGMs) in the abdominal musculature have been discussed in terms of their symptoms, activation mechanisms, and perpetuating factors. Trigger points in the abdominal region often overlap, making it difficult to attribute pain to specific muscles, such as the obliques and transverse abdominis. A banded pattern of pain is described across the abdomen, extending between the anterior costal borders and often concentrated at the xiphoid process. This pain can be provoked by PGMs in the cranial portion of the transverse abdominis, as well as by PGMs in the insertion zone of the lower costal cartilages, resulting in pain during breathing. PGMs of the transverse abdominis can cause myogenic inhibition and weakness in the muscle itself, which has been associated with various clinical conditions. Adequate activation of the transverse abdominis is crucial, especially in patients with persistent groin pain, as its weakness may contribute to chronic low back pain problems (80, 81, 83).

- PGMs in the abdominal region are related to several muscles, including: Rectus abdominis, abdominal oblique musculature, diaphragm, lumbar multifidus, serratus anterior, pelvic floor muscles, iliopsoas, hip adductors (80, 81, 83).
- Dry needling technique: For the treatment of PGMs in the transverse abdominal muscle, the use of superficial dry needling (DOT) in conjunction with conservative treatment is recommended. The variability in the muscle thickness of the three layers of the abdominal wall complicates the determination of a safe depth for deep SP, making the use of ultrasound-guided or EMG-guided puncture preferable when performing this technique (80, 81, 83).
- Risks and safety measures: To prevent complications, such as accidental introduction of the needle into the peritoneum, it is essential to take extreme antiseptic measures: strictly follow the rules of hygiene during the procedure and perform the puncture according to established procedures to ensure patient safety and avoid infection (80, 81, 83).

5.3. PS for thigh musculature.

5.3.1. Sartorio.

- Examination of the PGMs: The evaluation of trigger points (PGMs) in the sartorius muscle is performed by flat palpation with the patient in the supine position. This muscle can present PGMs along its entire length due to its non-aligned tendon intersections, so it is essential to explore its entire length. Unlike other PGMs, those of the sartorius usually cause superficial pain that is described as unpleasant and stabbing, and may also refer to superficial tingling or burning sensations. Once located and treated, it is essential to avoid sustained shortening of the sartorius, which can occur when sitting in positions such as the lotus or sleeping in the fetal position. Any significant lower limb dysmetria should also be corrected. Self-application techniques for pressure release or transverse friction massage can be taught, as these techniques do not limit mobility, unlike muscle stretching (84).

- Association with other PGMs: PGMs of the sartorius do not usually occur in isolation and are frequently associated with PGMs in other muscles (84).
    - Proximal: Related to the rectus femoris. Proximally, sartorius PGMs may be related to meralgia paresthetica, a condition caused by entrapment of the lateral femoral cutaneous nerve as it passes through taut bands of the sartorius. Symptoms include paresthesias and dysesthesias in the anterolateral aspect of the thigh, which may extend to the knee. This condition is more common in patients with abdominal overweight or in pregnant women.
    - Media: Associated with the hip adductors, especially in soccer players with pubalgia or in patients with problems in the coxofemoral joint.
    - Distal: They are frequently associated with a diagnosis of goose foot tendinopathy or with degenerative pathologies in the tibiofemoral joint, especially in valgus deformities of the knee.
- Dry needling: To treat PGMs of the sartorius muscle, prior treatment of PGMs in related muscles is recommended. The patient should be supine with the hip and knee in neutral position. If the muscle is very tight, a small pillow can be placed under the knee to facilitate palpation of the proximal insertion of the sartorius (84).
    - Palpation: The muscle should be palpated along its course, looking for tight bands and their corresponding PGMs.
    - Needle Choice: In thin patients, a 0.25 mm x 25 mm needle directed perpendicular to the taut band is used. For patients with more adipose panniculus, a 0.25 mm x 40 mm or longer needle is recommended, making sure that the needle passes through the adipose panniculus before inserting it into the muscle.

- Muscle Contraction: To improve the perception of the muscle barrier, the patient can be asked to maintain a gentle contraction of the muscle until he/she feels contact with it.

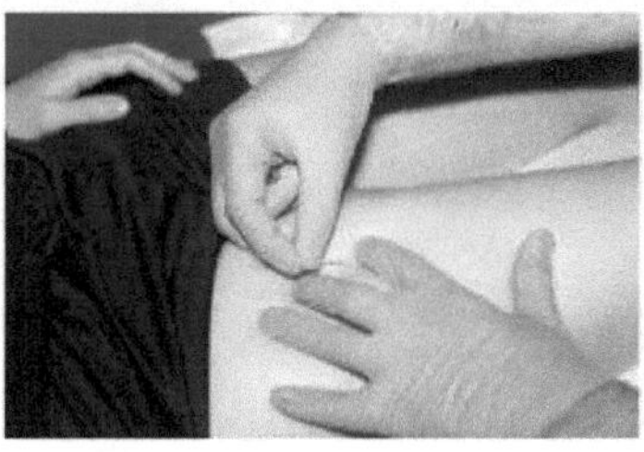

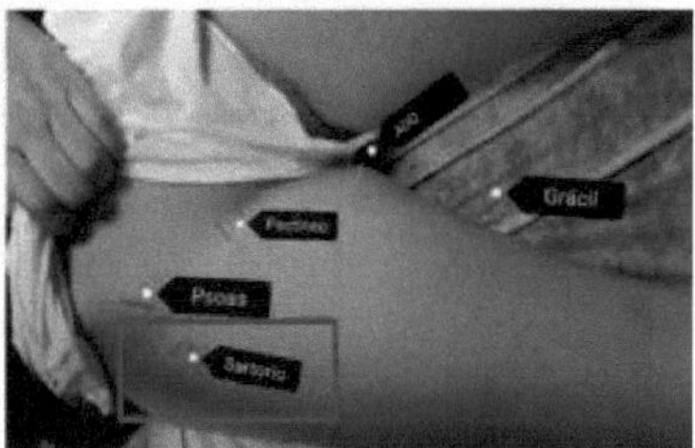

Figure 23. PS in PGM of the sartorius (54).

- Hazards and precautions (84):
  - Femoral neurovascular bundle: It is located on the medial aspect of the thigh, so accidental puncture should be avoided by not introducing the needle deeper than 20 mm.
  - Lateral femoral cutaneous nerve: This nerve crosses the sartorius in its proximal area, so care should be taken when inserting the needle in that area.
  - If the needle touches any branch, the patient may feel an electrical sensation in the anterolateral aspect of the thigh, in which case the needle should be withdrawn and its direction modified.

5.3.2. Quadriceps femoris.

Most knee dysfunctions are associated with a myofascial component that accompanies various structural elements that cause pain. According to Baldry, the lower extremity muscles that most frequently develop active myofascial trigger points (MTPs) are those of the quadriceps femoris. Overloading these muscles may activate MTrPs or, alternatively, these may be secondary to alterations in the knee, hip, ankle or foot that modify gait (85, 86).

- Causes of PGM activation in the quadriceps (85, 86):

- Muscle overload: Often related to sports activities, mountaineering, jumping, kneeling, squatting, carrying heavy objects or wearing high heels. Overload can arise especially from vigorous eccentric contractions or attempts to strengthen the muscle with loads close to the ankle.
- Surgical interventions: knee procedures that may contribute to PGM activation in the quadriceps.
- Immobilization: Orthopedic problems that require immobilization of the knee, which may result in the formation of PGMs.
- Direct injuries: Concussions or injections of drugs into the muscle are direct aggressions that can cause the formation of PGMs.
- Quadriceps PGMs can alter patellar mechanics and hinder knee mobility, being one of the main causes of knee pain of myofascial origin. Some diagnosed conditions, such as "jumper's knee" or "runner's knee," may actually be quadriceps referred pain.

- Quadriceps PGMs are associated with several clinical conditions, such as: anterior knee pain, patellofemoral pain syndrome, quadriceps tendinopathy, "jumper's knee", iliotibial band friction syndrome, meniscopathies, osteoarthritis/arthritis of the knee, chondropathies, phantom limb pain, bursitis and "growing pains" (85, 86).
- Symptoms of PGMs in the quadriceps, PGMs in the quadriceps can cause: anterior, lateral and medial pain in the knee, this pain can extend distally to the thigh and weakness and increased muscle tension or shortening of the quadriceps, which can be confused with other pathologies such as tendinopathies or bursitis (85, 86).
- Treatment: It is essential to recognize that treatment of knee dysfunction will not be successful if it is assumed that the problem is located only in the knee joint. It is essential to explore the various quadriceps fascicles for PGMs. If these are not treated, the patient will not progress adequately with strengthening exercises, stretching and functional recovery. Identification and treatment of

PGMs are crucial, because if these PGMs are left untreated, they can perpetuate tightness in related muscles, such as the hamstrings, even in a latent state. This can lead to a cycle of pain and weakness that prevents effective patient recovery (85, 86).

5.3.3. Rectus femoris.

The rectus femoris, being a muscle with a bipenniform architecture, presents a particular distribution of myofascial trigger points (MTrPs) that can be located almost anywhere in the muscle. It is not uncommon for the same patient to present multiple MTrPs in different areas of the rectus femoris (85, 86).

- Preferential PGM locations: There are preferential locations for these PGMs, the most common being (85, 86):
  - Proximally in the thigh: Just below the anteroinferior iliac spine. This location is associated with deep anterior thigh and inner knee pain. The patient usually describes the pain as localized below and around the patella.
  - Near the knee: Sometimes PGMs are located just above the knee, causing local and deep pain. This distal PGM may be associated with PGMs in the vastus lateralis.
- Rectus femoris PGMs can generate several symptoms, including (85, 86):
  - Nocturnal pain: This pain may awaken the patient during the night.
  - Deep pain on the inside of the knee: A common symptom that can be described as intense and local.
  - Weakness when descending stairs: This feeling of weakness becomes more noticeable in activities that require descending, which may inhibit the patellar reflex response.
- Causes of PGM activation in the rectus femoris (85, 86):
  - Shortening Position: Sitting for long periods places the rectus femoris in a shortened position, favoring the appearance of PGM.

- Muscle Overload: Activities involving powerful or repetitive hip flexion, such as mountain climbing, cycling, running, fast walking, kicking a ball, swimming (especially fluttering), improper footwear (wearing high heels or soft soles can also contribute to the development of PGMs).
- Anomalous Hip Mechanics: Dysfunctions in the hip, as well as in cases of fractures or surgeries in this joint or in the knee, may result in PGM activation in the rectus femoris.

- Interaction with other muscles: PGMs in the iliopsoas, sartorius (proximally), and adjacent muscles may contribute to PGMs in the rectus femoris (85, 86).
- Lancing technique: Patient in supine position with the hip in neutral rotation and the knee in extension. Anatomical landmarks are located between the anterosuperior iliac spine and the superior border of the patella. A flat palpation of the muscle is performed to identify tight bands and sore spots. The patient can perform a hip flexion with the knee in extension to differentiate the rectus femoris from other muscles such as the sartorius. Use a 0.30 mm x 50 mm needle and direct it perpendicular to the tight band. If the needle reaches the bone, the rectus femoris and underlying vastus intermedius can be punctured (85, 86).

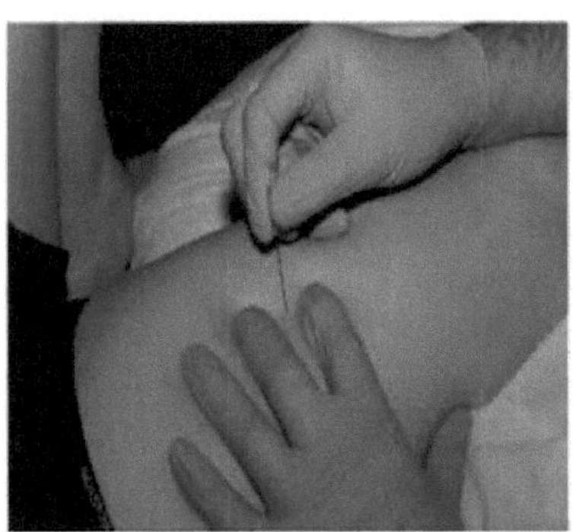

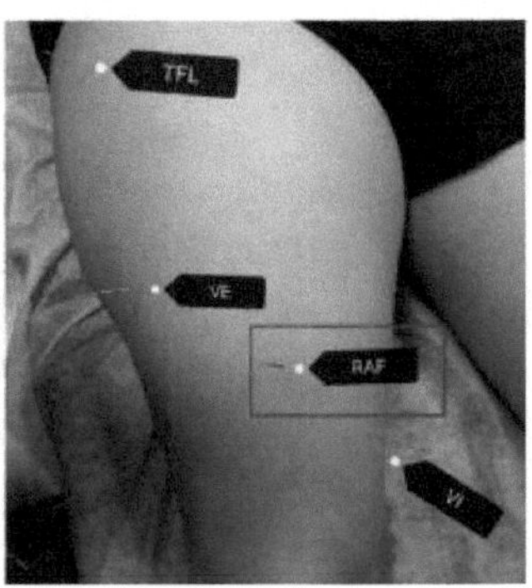

Figure 24. PS in PGM of the rectus femoris (54).

5.3.4. Vastus intermedius.

Myofascial trigger points (MTrPs) of the vastus intermedius have specific characteristics that are important to recognize for effective diagnosis and treatment (85, 86).

- Location of the PGMs: The PGMs of the vastus intermedius can be located at various heights along the muscle, but their most common location is approximately a few centimeters distal to the proximal area of the rectus femoris PGMs (85, 86).
- Underestimation of the PGMs: Many times, these PGMs are underestimated due to their location, since they are covered by the rectus femoris and cannot be palpated directly. This situation highlights the importance of selective palpation (SP), which is fundamental to differentiate between the vastus intermedius and rectus femoris (85, 86).
- Referred pain of the vastus intermedius PGMs is characterized by (85, 86):
    - Localization of pain: It is felt in the anterior and medial thigh, with a caudal spread from the PGM.
    - Movements that aggravate the pain: This pain usually manifests with movement of the knee and is infrequent at rest. It usually appears when walking and intensifies when climbing stairs.
    - Post-sedentary stiffness: After prolonged periods of sitting, the patient may experience difficulty in straightening the knee, which may result in limping.
    - Specific symptoms associated with vastus intermedius PGMs
    - Pain with knee motion: Motion activates the PGMs, resulting in significant pain.
    - Anterior thigh pain: The PGM is located within the painful area reported by the patient.
    - Lameness after prolonged sitting: Stiffness and pain after prolonged sitting can lead to difficulty walking properly.
- Relationship with other MMPs: vastus intermedius MMPs often do not occur in isolation, but are associated with other quadriceps MMPs, thus complicating the clinical picture. This means that

treatment must address all related PGMs to achieve effective recovery (85, 86).

- Lancing technique: with the patient in the supine position, the professional introduces the needle perpendicularly to the muscle surface and directly on the PG identified by flat palpation. Look for a sore spot on the anterolateral aspect of the thigh, palpating through or lateral to the rectus femoris. Use a 0.30 mm x 50 mm or 0.30 mm x 60 mm needle depending on the location of the PGMs or the patient's corpulence (85, 86).

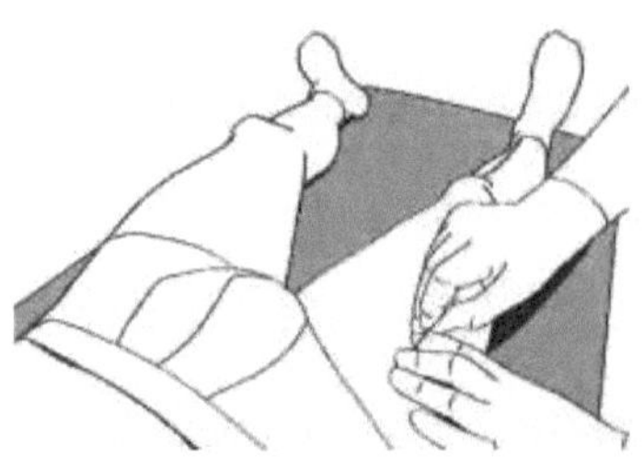
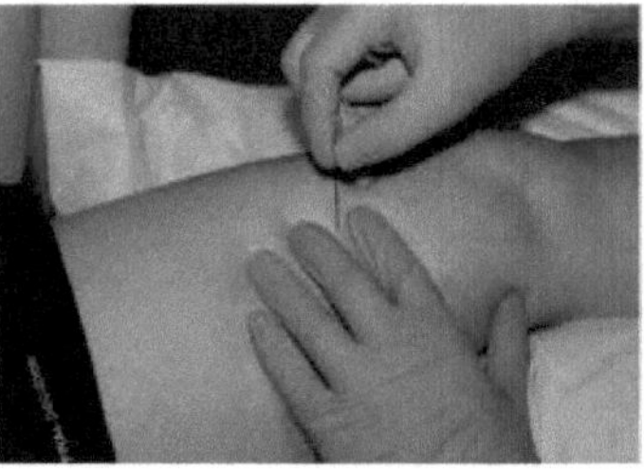

Figure 25. PS in PGM of the vastus intermedius (53, 54).

5.3.5. Lateral vastus.

Myofascial trigger points (MTrPs) in the vastus lateralis are a common source of pain affecting both the hip and knee. Their characteristics, symptoms and their impact on knee function are detailed below (85, 86).

- Location of the PGMs (85, 86):
  - Lateral hip and thigh pain: PGMs of this muscle can cause lateral hip and outer thigh pain.
  - Knee pain: They are a common source of knee pain, being the only anterior muscle that can cause pain in the back of this joint.
  - Patellar block: The PGMs located in the distal and anterior part of the vastus lateralis are responsible for patellar block, as well as pain at the lateral border of the patella, which sometimes extends up the lateral aspect of the thigh.

- Referred pain: PGMs in the distal region and posterior fibers may refer pain to the lateral aspect of the patella and more extensively to the lateral aspect of the thigh and leg.
- Covered by the iliotibial band: The part of the vastus lateralis is mainly covered by the iliotibial band, which makes it difficult to identify by palpation.
- Mid-thigh pain: In the mid-thigh area, at the posterior border of the vastus lateralis, PGMs have been identified that cause pain in the posterior lateral region of the thigh and in the lateral aspect of the popliteal fossa.
- Pain in the proximal region: In the medial thigh, PGMs in the central area can cause intense pain in the lateral aspect of the thigh, reaching almost to the iliac crest above and around the lateral border of the patella below.
- Insertional PGMs: PGMs have been described in the proximal end of the vastus lateralis, producing pain and hypersensitivity to local pressure.

- Associated symptoms (85, 86):
  - Pain in the lateral aspect of the knee and thigh: It presents as a sharp or dull pain in the lateral aspect, which may be constant or intermittent.
  - Patellar locking: Tight bands can cause lateral traction on the patella, hindering its movement and causing locking, especially when in slight flexion.
  - Growing pains in children: MGPs in the vastus lateralis are common in children, often associated with so-called "growing pains".
  - Difficulty walking: Walking can be painful if MMPs are active, and lying on the muscle can be uncomfortable, even disrupting sleep.
  - Effect on knee function: Weakness caused by the vastus medialis PGMs, in combination with tension of the vastus lateralis PGMs, may contribute to patellar imbalances and conditions such as patellofemoral pain syndrome and chondropathies.

- Activities that can trigger PGM (85, 86):
    - Overexertion: Any activity that involves considerable work on the legs, such as running, jumping, or high-intensity exercise, can predispose to the onset of MMPs.
    - Direct blows: A direct blow to the area can also activate PGM, as can holding the leg in an outstretched position for prolonged periods.
    - Immobilization: Any therapy that prevents knee flexion may perpetuate vastus lateralis PGMs.
- Puncture technique: for puncture of the PGs located in the anterior part of the vastus lateralis muscle, the patient is placed in the supine position. For puncture of the PGs located in the part of the muscle posterior to the iliotibial tract, the patient is placed in lateral decubitus. For distal PGMs in the anterior part, use a 0.25 mm x 40 mm needle, directed toward the bone. For distal PGMs in the posterior, use a 0.30 mm x 40 mm needle, also directed toward the bone.

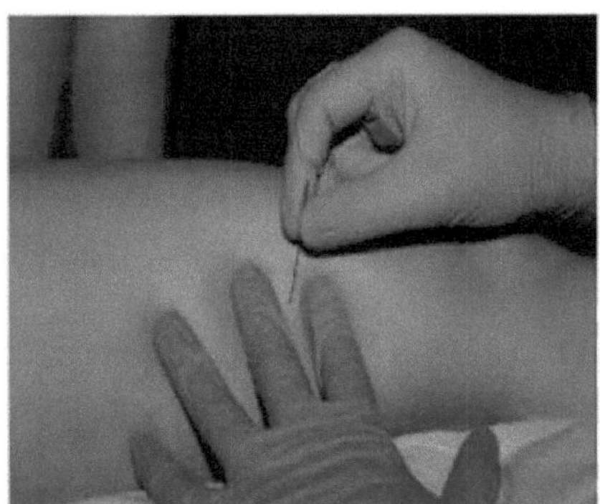

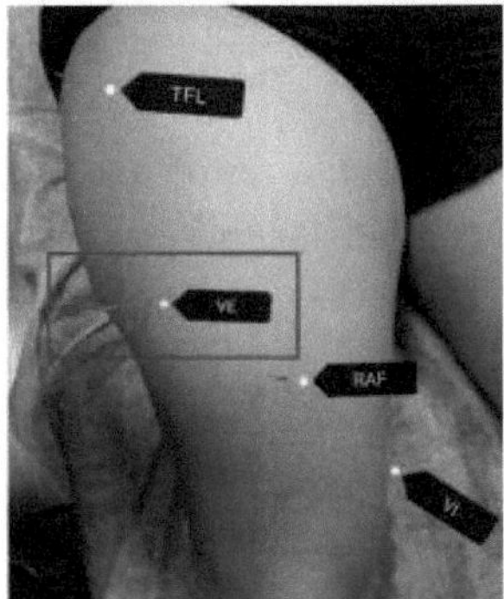

Figure 26. PS in PGM of the vastus lateralis (53, 54).

5.3.6. Vasto medialis.

Myofascial trigger points (MTrPs) in the vastus medialis can have a significant impact on knee function, causing pain and weakness.

Their characteristics, symptoms and how they can influence patient health are described below (85, 86).

- Location of the PGMs (85, 86):
    - Variable height: The vastus medialis PGMs can be found at different heights in the muscle:
    - Distal PGMs: Located a few centimeters above the patella, they are the most likely to refer pain in the anterior and medial part of the knee. This pain can cause sudden weakness in the knee, which can lead the patient to fall.
    - Proximal PGMs: Generally located in the medial part of the thigh, next to the adductor muscles. These can frequently accompany the distal PGMs, referring continuous pain in the middle and lower part of the thigh and in the anteromedial aspect of the knee.
- Associated symptoms (85, 86):
    - Insidious pain: vastus medialis PGMs may cause a dull ache that initially presents in the knee, and occasionally in the inner thigh. This pain may even awaken the patient during the night.
    - Diagnostic confusion: This myofascial pain is often confused with inflammatory joint processes, osteoarthritis, ligament injuries and tendinopathies, which can lead to misdiagnosis.
    - Knee weakness and failure: If not properly treated, PGMs can progress, causing episodes of quadriceps inhibition resulting in failure due to weakness during gait.
    - Constant tension: Mild but constant tension of the PGMs may contribute to the development of patellar tendinopathies, especially in their lower pole.
- Contributing factors (85, 86):
    - Muscle overload: Intense sports activities, such as running or deep squats, can overuse the quadriceps and overload the vastus medialis.
    - Aggressive physical therapy: stretching and strengthening exercises, especially in open kinetic chain with distal loads, can aggravate vastus medialis PGMs.

- Hyperpronation of the foot: Hyperpronation can overload this muscle and perpetuate its PGMs.
- Direct trauma: Direct blows to the knee are another frequent cause of PGM activation in the vastus medialis.

- Importance of diagnosis and treatment: It is crucial to perform a thorough examination for PGMs, as well as to treat any trigger points identified in the hip adductor, rectus femoris, vastus lateralis and tensor fascia lata muscles (85, 86).
- PS: With the patient in the supine position, the practitioner inserts the needle perpendicular to the muscle surface and directly over the PG identified by palpation. However, given the anatomical connections between the adductor magnus and adductor longus muscles, muscle stretching is best performed with the knee in flexion and the hip in abduction. Flat palpation is performed to locate tight bands and PGMs, which will be punctured using 0.25 mm x 40 mm needles. Due to severe pain during and after needling, it is recommended that dry electrostimulation be considered as an additional treatment technique (85, 86).

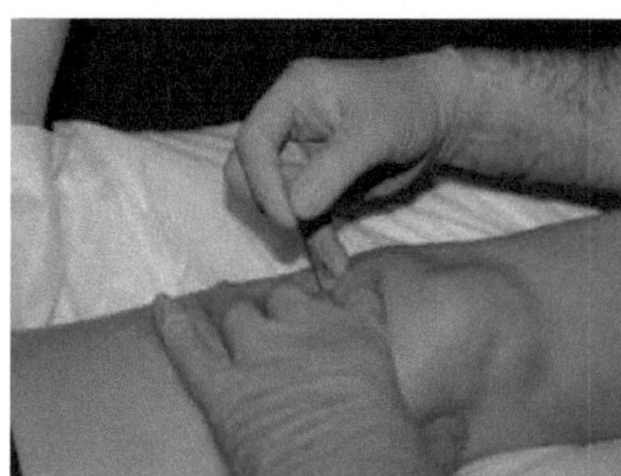

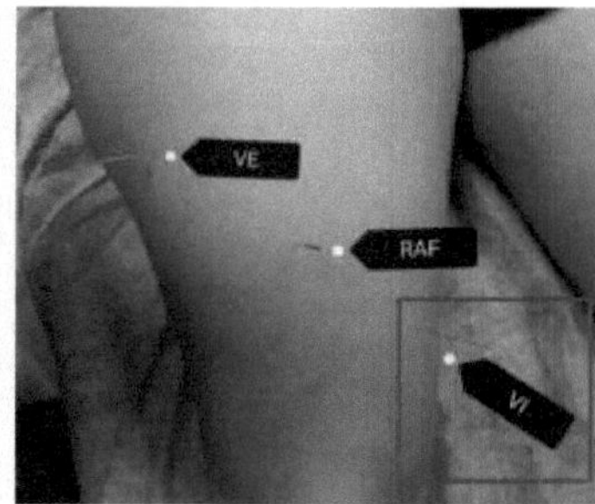

Figure 27. PS in PGM of the vastus medialis (54).

5.3.7. Semimembranosus.

- Location: Hamstring PGMs are usually found 8-12 cm from the knee flexor, in the distal part of the thigh. However, they can occur in various parts of these muscles (87, 88).
- Referred pain (87, 88):

- Semimembranosus: Pain radiates from the proximal part of the back of the thigh, in the region of the gluteal fold, and may extend towards the calf.
- Semitendinosus: shares the same pain distribution.
- Biceps femoris: Causes a duller pain compared to the other two.
- Patients may experience pain when walking, which can lead to limping. Compression of the hamstrings during rest may also cause pain in the buttock, back of the thigh and knee.

- Symptoms and misdiagnosis: Hamstring PGMs can cause symptoms similar to those of quadriceps PGMs, increasing tension and overloading this muscle. They are commonly mistaken for sciatica or hamstring tendinopathy due to the distribution of pain and associated stiffness (87, 88).
- Hamstring PGMs can be activated by (87, 88):
  - Muscle Injuries: These can arise from an injury, causing pain and decreased flexibility.
  - Posture: Keeping the knee bent for long periods of time (such as sitting) may contribute to the development of PGMs.
  - Sedentary Lifestyle: This negatively affects hamstring health.
  - Sports: Activities such as soccer, basketball and track and field, which require sudden accelerations, are prone to cause hamstring injuries.
  - Muscle Weakness: Weakness of the gluteus maximus or lateral hip rotators can lead to hamstring overload, having to compensate for this weakness.
- PS: Patient position in prone or supine decubitus. The aim is to identify the PGMs by flat or clamp palpation. A 0.30 mm x 50 mm or 0.30 mm x 60 mm needle is recommended, depending on the position and technique used (87, 88).

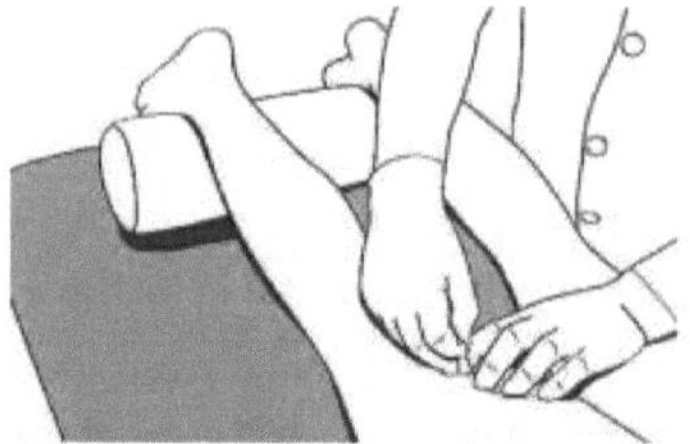 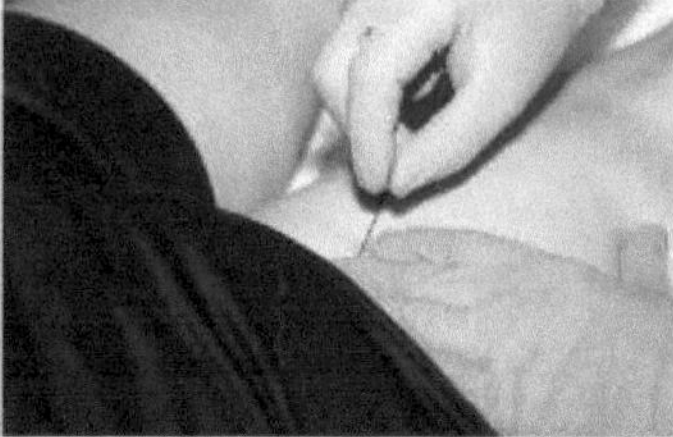

Figure 28. PS in PGM of the semimembranosus (53, 54).

- Precautions (87, 88):
  - Sciatic nerve: It is important to avoid contact with the sciatic nerve, which is located near the hamstring muscles. The direction of the needle must be precise so as not to compromise neurovascular structures.
  - Technique: The medial inclination of the needle reduces the risk of nerve injury.

5.3.8. Semitendinosus.

- The semitendinosus PGMs are commonly found between 8 cm and 12 cm from the knee flexure, in the medial part of the muscle. However, they can be located in other areas, especially in the proximal third, due to the innervation zones on both sides of the tendon intersection (87, 88).
- Referred pain: The pain provoked by the semitendinosus PGMs radiates mainly to the proximal area of the posterior thigh, in the region of the gluteal crease. The pain pattern may extend caudally down the posterior thigh, even reaching the calf. Compared to semimembranosus, semitendinosus pain is sharp and distinct, while biceps femoris pain tends to be more dull (87, 88).
- Symptoms and activation mechanisms: Semitendinosus PGMs present with symptoms similar to those of other hamstring muscles due to trigger point activation and their perpetuating mechanisms. Patients may experience pain on walking, stiffness and weakness in the affected region (87, 88).

- Dry needling: The dry needling technique for semitendinosus is performed in a similar manner to that for semimembranosus. It can be performed in prone or supine position, depending on clinician preference and patient comfort (87, 88).
- Precautions and hazards: As in the semimembranosus puncture, there is a risk of accidentally puncturing the sciatic nerve, which is located in the midline of the thigh, between the biceps femoris and the semimembranosus. Distally, in the popliteal fossa, there is also a risk of damaging the femoral blood vessels (87, 88).

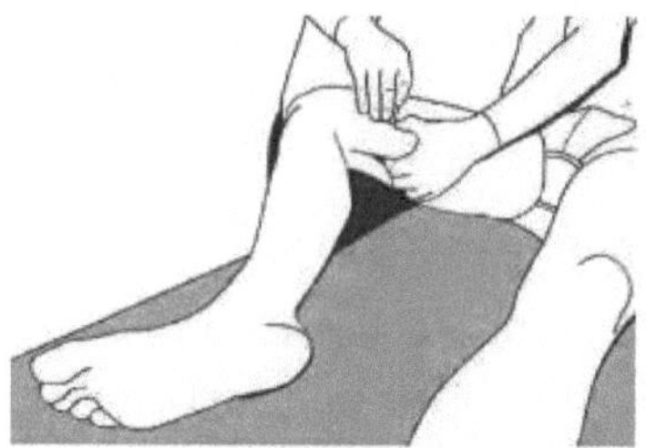
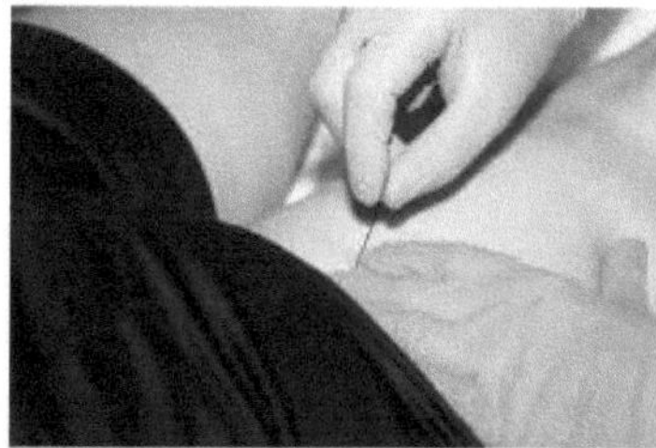

Figure 29. PS in PGM of the semitendinosus (53, 54).

5.3.9. Biceps femoris.

- Biceps femoris MMPs: Biceps femoris MMP pain is described as a dull ache that is localized behind the knee. This pain may radiate to the posterolateral aspect of the thigh and sometimes concentrate in the head of the fibula. In addition, the pain may extend into the upper thigh and into the calf. Biceps femoris PGMs may also cause nocturnal pain, disturbing the patient's sleep (87, 88).
- Symptoms and trigger mechanisms: Hamstring injuries are common among athletes, and the biceps femoris, especially its long head, is the most frequently injured muscle in this category. Symptoms include pain and stiffness in the back of the thigh, as well as possible decreased functionality during physical activities (87, 88).
- Dry needling: For dry needling of the PGMs of the biceps femoris, the patient should be in prone position with a small pillow under the feet to keep the knee in slight flexion. A flat palpation is

performed along the muscle to identify tender points and tight bands. Once the PGM is located, it is recommended to use a 0.30 mm x 50 mm needle, directing it anteromedially from the lateral part of the midline of the thigh to minimize the risk of contact with the sciatic nerve (87, 88).

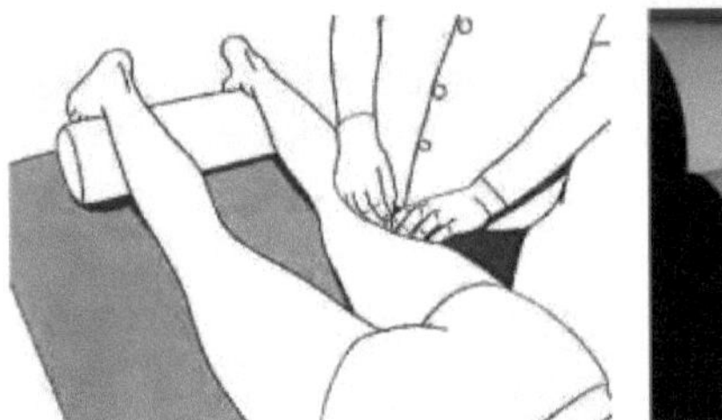
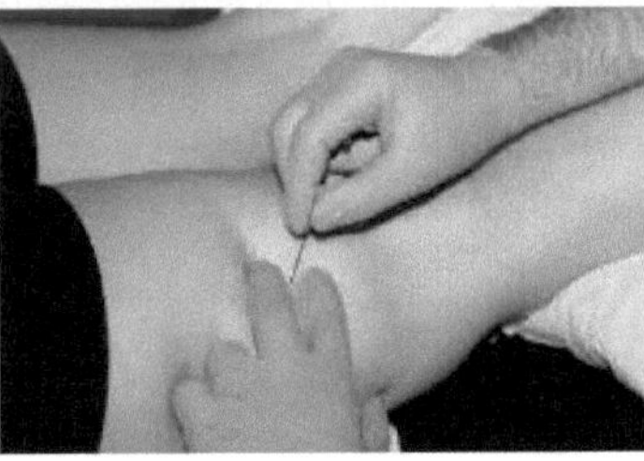

PS in PGM of the biceps femoris (53, 54).

- Dangers and Precautions: The sciatic nerve lies between the ischial tuberosity and the greater trochanter in the proximal thigh, and travels approximately along the midline of the thigh, between the biceps femoris and semimembranosus. Distally, branches of the sciatic nerve, as well as the tibial nerve and the peroneal nerve, lie between the semimembranosus and the biceps femoris tendon. In the popliteal fossa, the femoral vessels are located close to the sciatic nerve. By following the above indications for needle direction, the risk of contact with neurovascular structures is significantly reduced, but the precautions detailed in the corresponding chapter on punctures should be followed (87, 88).

5.3.10. Pectineus.

- Location: The pectineus PGMs are located just below the superior pubic ramus, accessible by palpation in the space between the femoral vein and the adductor longus tendon (89).
- Pain: They cause a deep pain in the groin, which may present as a sharp pain or a continuous dull ache. This pain sometimes feels as if it originates in the hip joint (89).

- Irradiation: Pain may spread over the anteromedial aspect of the thigh, superiorly, and distribute over the proximal insertion zone of the adductor magnus. It is uncommon for pain to occur in isolation, as it is often associated with PGMs in other adductors or in the iliopsoas (89).
- Mobility: Although it may restrict hip separation, it is generally other adductors that limit joint mobility the most (89).
- Activation mechanisms: The mechanisms of activation of the pectineus PGMs are common to other adductors. This includes factors such as overuse, maintained postures or activities involving repeated contraction of the muscle. In relation to the adductor magnus, it is recommended that information on its activation be consulted to better understand the associated mechanisms (89).
- Dry needling: For dry needling of the pectineus pectoralis PGMs, the patient should be in supine decubitus with the hip in slight lateral rotation and the knee in extension. The approach route is between the femoral vessels and the adductor longus tendon. It is suggested to locate the sartorius as a reference, and then palpate the anatomical structures of the region, moving from lateral to medial until reaching the pectineus, which is located lateral to the adductor longus tendon. It is crucial to locate the femoral pulse to avoid accidental puncture of the femoral vessels. The muscle is explored by flat palpation to locate tight bands and sore spots. Once the PGM is identified, a 0.25 mm x 40 mm needle is used and directed perpendicular to the tight band. However, due to the depth of the muscle, it is recommended to use a longer needle, 50 mm or 60 mm, to reach adjacent areas such as the adductor brevis and the upper part of the adductor magnus (89).

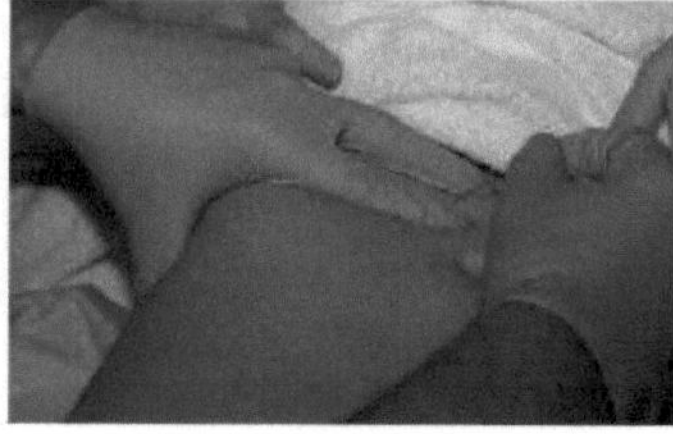

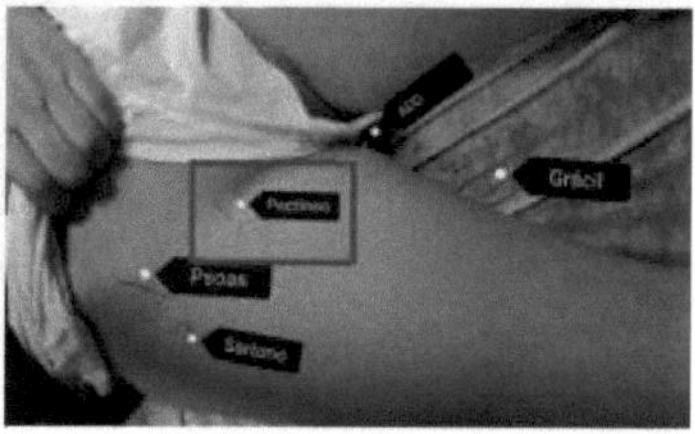

Figure 31. PS in PGM of the pectineus (54).

- Hazards and precautions (89):
  - Femoral neurovascular bundle: The femoral neurovascular bundle is located on the medial aspect of the thigh, over the pectineus. Before performing the puncture, the femoral pulse should be located and at least one finger should be kept at a distance as a safety measure.
  - Risks in Deep Punctures: If an attempt is made to explore the short and minimus adductors, there is a risk of affecting the branches of the obturator nerve and the medial femoral circumflex artery, which is a branch of the deep femoral artery. The precautions established in the corresponding chapter should be followed to avoid complications.

5.3.11. Adductor magnus.

- Location: The PGMs of the adductor magnus are located in the middle third of the thigh, just above the junction of the sartorius with the adductor longus, and very close to the femur. Although they may correspond to the ischiochondyle division of the muscle, they are commonly located in its lateral division (90, 91, 92).
- Referred pain: These PGMs may cause pain radiating from the groin along the medial aspect of the thigh to the knee. The pain pattern does not always manifest completely and often presents as a deep groin pain. Because of their deep location, they are often an overlooked cause of persistent groin pain (90, 91, 92).
- Other locations: PGMs have been identified near the proximal insertion of the adductor magnus at the ischial tuberosity, which may cause diffuse, poorly localized pain in the pelvis. This pain may be acute and localized to areas such as the pubis, vagina, rectum, prostate or bladder. This intrapelvic pain may be confused with visceral, urologic or gynecologic problems, and may intensify during sexual intercourse (90, 91, 92).
- The adductor magnus PGMs can be activated by various factors, such as (90, 91, 92):

- Injury: An unexpected slip or fall can cause a sudden contraction or overstretching of the adductor muscles.
- Sports activities: Exercises that require a large opening of the hips (such as gymnastics, running, or skiing) can overload the adductor musculature.
- Poor technique: Improper technique in activities such as cycling, where the knee moves medially, can lead to adductor overload.
- Prolonged sitting: Prolonged sitting, especially with the legs crossed, causes a sustained shortening of the adductor musculature.
- Footwear: High-heeled shoes and lower extremity dysmetria may also contribute to the activation of these PGMs.
- Surgical interventions: Hip surgery can activate PGMs and result in persistent postsurgical pain.
- Pathological conditions: Arthrosis of the coxofemoral joint and fractures of the femoral neck are common causes of PGM activation in this area.

- Symptoms: Pain presents as medial thigh and deep intrapelvic pain, often accompanied by tightness and weakness in the adductor muscles. It is common for patients to have difficulty finding a comfortable sleeping position (90, 91, 92).
- Dry needling: To treat the PGMs of the adductor magnus, the patient should be in homolateral lateral decubitus, with the hip and knee of the affected side flexed. The PGM is located in the middle third of the adductor magnus, which is above the sartorius, dorsal to the adductor longus and covered by the gracilis. It should be palpated with the thumb as flat as possible to identify a painful point on pressure. A 0.30 mm x 75 mm needle (or 60 mm in thin muscles) is used directed towards the femur, crossing the gracil on the surface. The needle can be angled slightly backward to explore the dorsal portion of the muscle, but avoid directing it excessively in that direction so as not to contact the sciatic nerve. To treat more proximal PGMs, the ischial tuberosity is used as a reference, palpating the proximal part of the adductor magnus and directing a

0.30 mm x 50 mm needle toward the tender points. This procedure can also be performed in prone position (90, 91, 92).

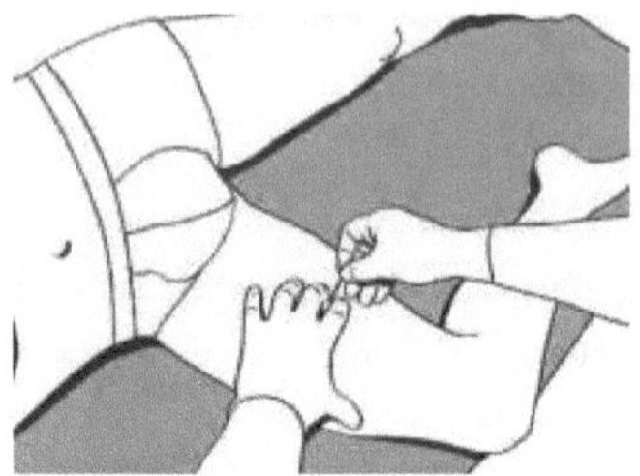
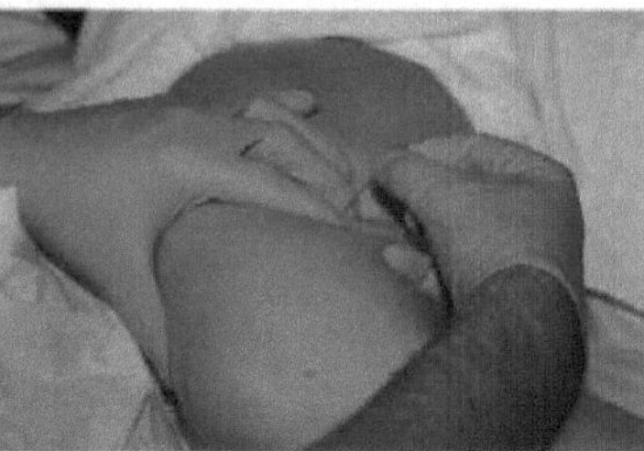

Figure 32. PS in PGM of the adductor magnus (53, 54).

- Hazards and precautions: During puncture of the central PGMs of the adductor magnus, it is crucial to avoid excessive angulations of the needle in the dorsal direction to prevent accidental contact with the sciatic nerve (90, 91, 92).

5.3.12. Adductor long and short.

- Location: The PGMs of the adductor longus and adductor brevis are usually found in their most proximal portion. Since the adductor longus covers the adductor brevis, palpation of the adductor brevis should be performed through the adductor longus.
- Referred pain: No clear distinction has been established between the referred pain patterns of both muscles. However, it is recognized that PGMs of these muscles are one of the most frequent causes of groin pain. The pain is felt deep within the groin and may extend into the anteromedial aspect of the thigh and leg. Clinical experience supports that groin pain is an essential component of referred pain from these PGMs. In addition, these trigger points may restrict hip mobility (90, 91, 92).
- Other manifestations: PGMs may refer pain to the superior and anteromedial aspect of the knee, as well as be associated with vastus medialis PGMs in cases of anterior knee pain or femoropatellar pain syndrome. Pain may extend down the anteromedial aspect of the tibia (90, 91, 92).

- Symptoms: At rest, the pain tends to disappear, but there may be limitation in hip abduction and lateral rotation (90, 91, 92).
- The mechanisms of activation of the PGMs of the long and short adductors are similar to those of other adductors and are described in the section on adductor magnus. They generally include (90, 91, 92):
    - Trauma or Injury: Falls or overloads can activate these trigger points.
    - Repetitive Movements: Activities that require repetitive adduction or rotational movements may contribute to activation.
    - Prolonged Positions: Being in postures that favor the contraction of these muscles can provoke their activation.
- Symptoms: Deep groin and proximal groin pain, pain in and above the knee, restriction of hip abduction, and weakness. Related muscles include the adductors, abductors, and iliopsoas (90, 91, 92).
- Dry needling: To explore the adductor longus for tight bands, the patient should be in the supine position with the hip and knee flexed and the foot resting on the table. The physical therapist stands in a position homolateral to the thigh to be treated and drops the patient's knee on his or her abdomen. The patient's leg should be relaxed in hip flexion with slight abduction. The tendon of this muscle is located and explored along its length by flat palpation, moving the fingers in an anteroposterior direction to identify tight bands with painful points. A 0.25 mm x 40 mm needle is used perpendicular to the most painful point of the localized tight band, directed towards the femur. If palpated in forceps, the needle is directed anteroposteriorly towards the fingers. Positioning the patient comfortably, with the hip in neutral position, simultaneous puncture of the adductor longus and adductor brevis can be performed, locating their PGMs by flat palpation and inserting a 0.30 mm x 50 mm needle perpendicular to the adductor longus, in

an anteroposterior direction. This technique is useful to approach both muscles at the same time (90, 91, 92).

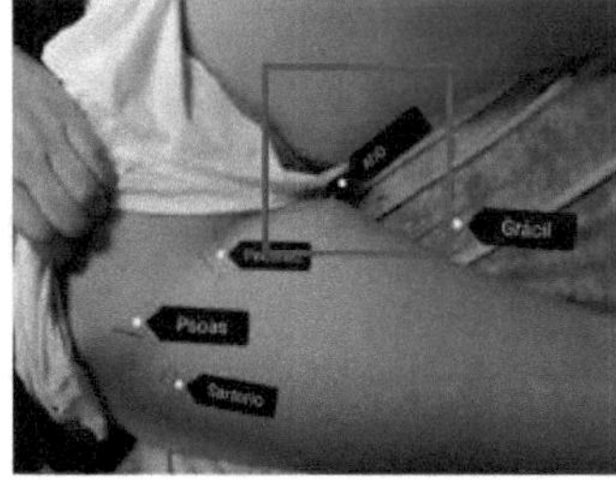

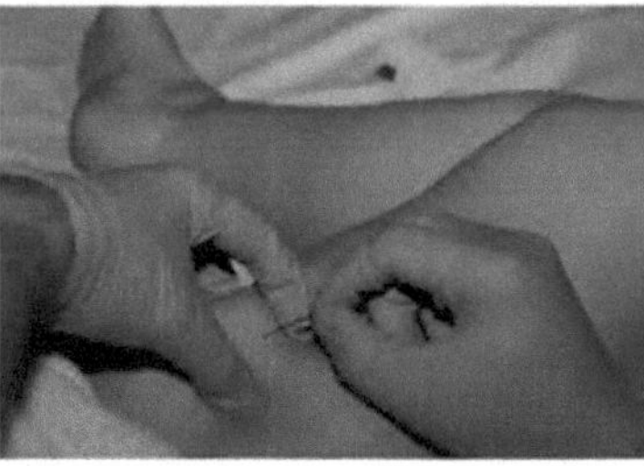

Figure 33. PS in PGM of the long and short adductor (54).

- Dangers and precautions: The femoral neurovascular bundle is located on the medial aspect of the thigh over the pectineus muscle. Before puncturing any muscle in this region, the femoral pulse should be located and a distance of at least one finger should be maintained as a safety distance when puncturing the adductors. The needle should never be directed toward the femoral pulse during puncture of the pectineus or the adductor longus and adductor brevis to avoid injury (90, 91, 92).

5.3.13. Graceful.

- Localization: PGMs of the gracilis can be found anywhere in the muscle, although they are commonly located in its proximal half (90, 91, 92).
- Referred pain: Unlike other muscles, the pain is local and not referred at a distance. It is described as a stabbing, burning pain under the skin, although it can also manifest as a more diffuse pain. This pain may be constant, even at rest, although walking usually relieves it (90, 91, 92).
- The mechanisms of activation of the PGMs of the gracilis are similar to those of other adductors, including (90, 91, 92):
    - Direct Trauma: Injuries or falls affecting the thigh region.

    - Repetitive Movements: Activities involving adduction or repetitive movements of the hip.
    - Prolonged postures: Being in positions that favor the contraction of the gracilis muscle can activate the PGMs.
- Symptoms: The pain is superficial and local, meaning that it is not felt in distant areas. This may make it difficult to identify the source of pain in some cases (90, 91, 92).
- Related muscles: adductors and iliopsoas (90, 91, 92).
- Dry needling: The patient should be in the supine position with the hip flexed and the foot resting on the examination table. The gracilis muscle is located immediately posterior to the adductor longus and can be easily palpated in forceps. Distally, the gracilis is located anterior to the semitendinosus, where it can also be palpated with forceps. A painful pressure point is sought within the area where the patient feels pain to identify a PGM. A 0.25 mm x 40 mm needle is used, directing it in an anteroposterior direction toward the fingers on the other side of the clamp (90, 91, 92).

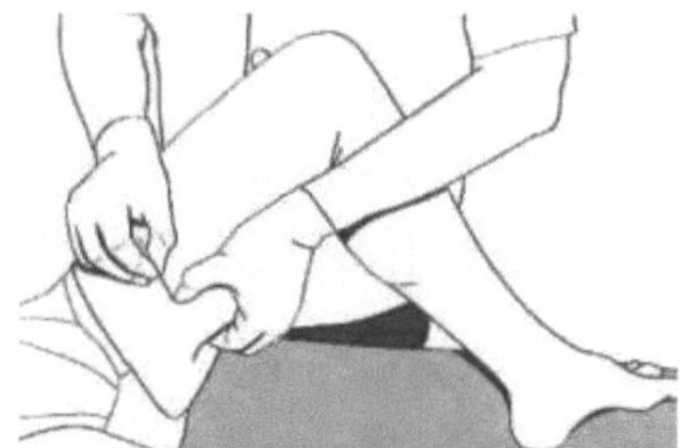

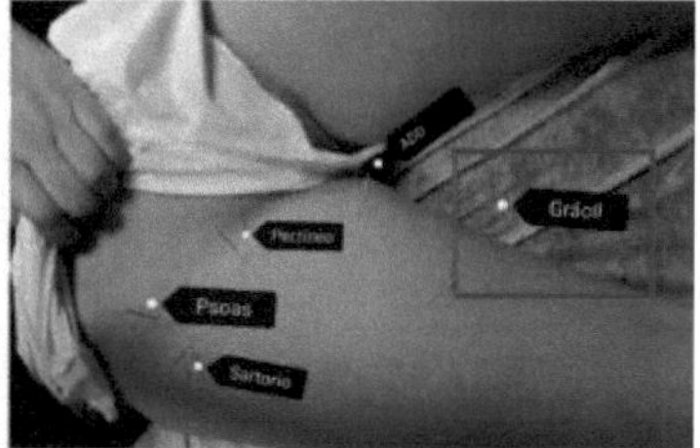

Figure 34. PS in PGM of the adductor gracilis (53).

- Hazards and precautions: No special recommendations or outstanding hazards are described for lancet puncture. However, it is essential to follow general aseptic and disinfection measures when performing any puncture procedure (90, 91, 92).

5.3.14. Puncture of other structures (PGNM).

In all the above-mentioned cases, aseptic and disinfection measures should be maximized, especially due to the risk that the needle may contact the joint capsule and enter the circulation. This is crucial to prevent complications related to infection or vascular damage (93, 94, 95, 96, 97, 98):

- Peroneal collateral ligament: A ligamentous PGM is described in this ligament, which refers pain to the lateral part of the knee. It can be treated by superficial puncture, deep puncture or dry electro-puncture.
- Collateral ligaments of the knee: Baldry mentions PG in the proximal and distal insertions of these ligaments, suggesting their deactivation by dry needling (PS).
- Infrapatellar fat pad (Hoffa's fat): PG can be found in this structure, and its treatment by superficial PS is recommended.
- Iliotibial girdle: PGs along the lateral aspect of the thigh can be treated with PS. Baldry suggests superficial PS, while Gunn recommends local deep PS.

5.4. PS for leg and foot musculature.

5.4.1. Popliteal.

- Localization: The central PGMs of the popliteus muscle are inaccessible to palpation. However, palpation of an insertional PGM on the posteromedial aspect of the tibia may indicate the presence of the central PGM (99, 100).
- Referred pain: It is mainly located in the posterior part of the knee. However, according to the clinical experience of the authors, variations are observed that include pain in the posteromedial part of the tibia and in the anteromedial aspect, heading towards the goose foot area (99, 100).
- Symptoms (99, 100):
    - Difficulty moving the knee: Patients often complain of difficulty in fully extending the knee during the swing phase (stiffness) or flexing it when squatting.
    - Stiffness: This stiffness may manifest when getting out of bed in the morning or getting up from a chair after sitting for a while.

- Pain when descending slopes: Pain associated with popliteus muscle PGMs is intensified when descending slopes and wearing heels. Generally, there is no pain at rest.

- Activation mechanisms (99, 100):
  - Eccentric overload: The most common mechanism of PGM activation in the popliteus muscle is the eccentric overload that occurs due to internal rotation of the femur over the tibia in closed chain.
  - Joint problems: Other indirect mechanisms include problems in the knee joint, such as meniscopathies, hydroarthrosis and osteoarthritis.
- Related muscles: The most important muscles that can be influenced include the biceps femoris, vastus lateralis quadriceps and gastrocnemius (99, 100).
- Dry needling: The patient should be in lateral decubitus on the affected side, with the hip and knee flexed at 90°. The muscle was palpated just behind the proximal third of the tibia, laterally displacing the medial gastrocnemius to find an insertional PGM corresponding to the popliteus muscle. A 0.25 mm x 40 mm or, more commonly, 0.30 mm x 50 mm needle is recommended. The puncture is initiated by directing the needle towards the posterior aspect of the tibia. The central PGM is then sought by directing the needle laterally with a slight anterocranial tilt, keeping it close to the posterior aspect of the tibia or even contacting the bone (99, 100).

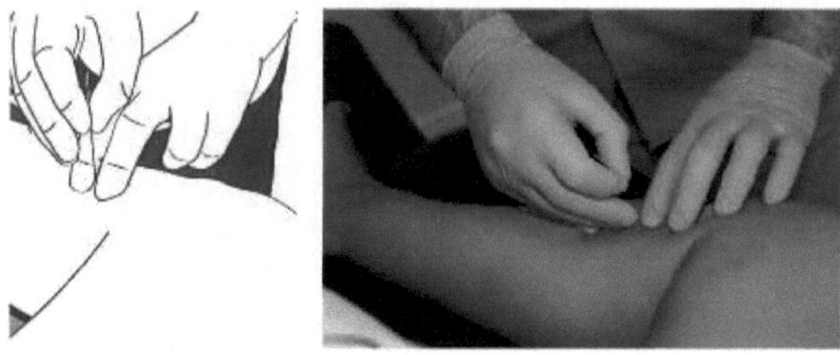

Figure 35. PS in popliteal PGM (53, 54).

- Hazards and precautions (99, 100):
  - Avoid puncture of the neurovascular bundle: It is crucial to avoid accidental puncture of the neurovascular bundle located in the midline of the posterior aspect of the leg, just behind the popliteus muscle.
  - General rules: In addition to following the general rules described for these situations, the needle should be kept very close to the posterior aspect of the tibia, using the contact with the bone as a reference.
  - Saphenous nerve branches: Some branches of the saphenous nerve may be present superficially in the area of needle insertion. If the needle contacts a nerve, the patient may experience a superficial electrical sensation on the inside of the leg. In this case, the needle should be removed and reinserted a few millimeters away.

5.4.2. Gastrocnemius.

- PGMs in the gastrocnemius muscle usually produce localized pain, although broader patterns affecting the posterior aspect of the lower limb may occur. PGMs in the medial head tend to reflect pain in the sole of the foot, especially in the area of the internal plantar arch, and sometimes the pain extends to the popliteal fossa and posterior aspect of the leg and ankle. In addition to pain, patients may experience cramping in the calf, particularly with PGMs in the central area of both heads. Pain in the back of the knee has also been noted to intensify when walking on sloping surfaces. The presence of PGMs in the gastrocnemius has been shown to have a direct relationship to intermittent claudication and it has been noted that treatment of these trigger points can improve symptoms without the need for circulatory changes (99, 100).
- Clinical symptoms: Localized and posterior knee pain when walking on inclined surfaces. Cramps in the calf (99, 100).
- Mechanisms of activation: The most common direct mechanism of PGM activation in the gastrocnemius is mechanical overload, either

from walking or running uphill, or from activities requiring powerful plantar flexion with the knee flexed. Other factors such as prolonged immobilization and joint problems in the knee and ankle may also contribute to its activation (99, 100).

- Dry needling (99, 100):
    - Popliteus muscle: The patient should be in lateral decubitus with the hip and knee flexed at 90º. Palpate the muscle behind the proximal third of the tibia and look for the insertional PGM. It is recommended to use a 0.25 mm x 40 mm or 0.30 mm x 50 mm needle, starting the treatment in the insertional PGM and then looking for the central PGM.
    - Gastrocnemius muscle: The patient should be in prone position, keeping the knee in semi-flexion. The PGMs can be located by palpation and puncture can be performed with needles of different calibers depending on the location of the PGM.

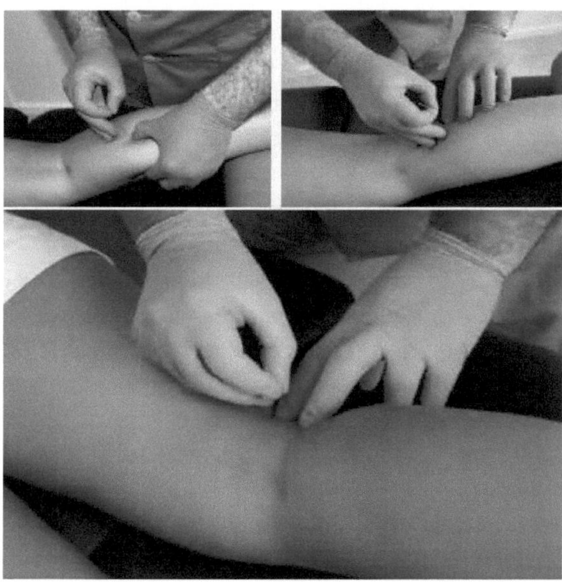

Figure 36. PS in PGM of the gastrocnemius (medial head, lateral head and lateral head proximal part) (54).

- Hazards and precautions (99, 100):
  - Popliteus muscle: Avoid accidental puncture of the neurovascular bundle, which is located in the midline of the posterior aspect of the leg. It is important to keep the needle close to the posterior aspect of the tibia and use the contact with the bone as a reference.
  - Gastrocnemius muscle: The sciatic nerve divides into the tibial and common peroneal nerves in the posterior thigh. The proximal anatomy causes the PGMs in the most proximal portions of the gastrocnemius to be proximal to the neurovascular bundle, requiring careful palpation.

5.4.3. Planting.

- Trigger points and referred pain: The most common referred pain from myofascial trigger points (MTrPs) in the plantar muscle is located primarily at the back of the knee. It may also extend downward to the mid-calf. Sometimes the pain can radiate to the sole of the foot and the base of the big toe, although it is unclear whether this extension is due to a PGM of the plantaris muscle or one in the lateral head of the gastrocnemius (99, 100).
- Dry needling: Because the plantaris muscle is covered by the lateral head of the gastrocnemius, the dry needling technique is the same as that used for that part of the gastrocnemius muscle (99, 100).
- Dangers and precautions: It is important to avoid puncture of the popliteal vessels and the tibial and peroneal nerves. To this end, the same precautions indicated for dry puncture of the proximal gastrocnemius areas should be followed and care should be taken with the proximity of neurovascular and articular structures (99, 100).

5.4.4. Oil.

- PGMs in the soleus muscle are located mainly in its medial and lateral part, and can cause different types of referred pain. The most common PGMs are located medially, causing pain in the Achilles tendon and heel, similar to plantar fasciitis or heel spurs. PGMs laterally and superiorly can cause deep calf pain, which may be mistaken for thrombophlebitis. Referred pain to the sacroiliac joint, the heel and even, in rare cases, to the jaw has also been observed (99, 100).
- Pain caused by soleus PGMs is associated with walking difficulties, especially when climbing stairs or slopes, and is sometimes accompanied by edema in the foot or ankle due to impaired venous pumping. These PGMs may also limit dorsal flexion of the ankle and weaken the soleus reflex (99, 100).
- They are often activated by acute or chronic overloads, such as running or slips, and may be related to other muscles such as the gluteus minimus or hamstrings (99, 100).
- Dry needling: To treat these PGMs by dry needling, 0.30 mm x 40 mm needles are used. The patient can be in prone or lateral decubitus, depending on the location of the PGM. The technique consists of palpating the muscle with a forceps and guiding the needle between the fingers that fix the PGM. Special precautions should be taken to avoid damaging the tibial nerve and tibial arteries or veins, especially when treating PGMs in the medial soleus area (99, 100).

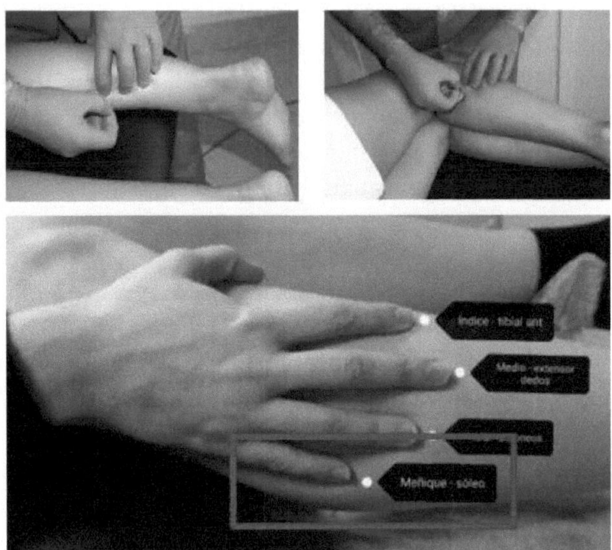

Figure 37. PS in PGM of the soleus (54).

5.4.5. Flexor digitorum longus.

- PGMs in the flexor digitorum longus muscle usually cause referred pain in the medial aspect of the sole of the foot, especially proximal to the triphalangeal toes. This pain may include the medial aspect of the ankle and calf, but rarely affects the heel. PGMs in this muscle may be related to diagnoses such as plantar fasciitis and residual pain after an ankle sprain. Although toe cramps are more commonly associated with the intrinsic flexors, in some cases flexor digitorum longus PGMs can also trigger them. Affected individuals often experience pain in the sole of the foot and toes when walking, which may lead to the use of orthopedic inserts (101, 102).
- These PGMs are activated by acute or chronic overloads, such as running, especially if there is hyperpronation of the foot. The use of inappropriate footwear, especially with stiff soles, can perpetuate these PGMs (101, 102).

- Dry needling: To perform dry needling, the patient is placed in lateral decubitus with the hip and knee flexed at 90º. The trigger point is located by flat palpation on the posteromedial aspect of the tibia, away from the soleus and medial gastrocnemius muscles. Once the PGM is located, a 0.25 mm x 40 mm needle is inserted in an anterolateral direction, keeping it close to or in contact with the posterior aspect of the tibia as a reference (101, 102).
- Dangers and precautions: It is important to avoid touching the neurovascular bundle (tibial nerve and posterior tibial and peroneal vessels), which is lateral to the muscle. To avoid complications, it is recommended to use the posterior aspect of the tibia as a reference, keeping the needle close to this structure (101, 102).

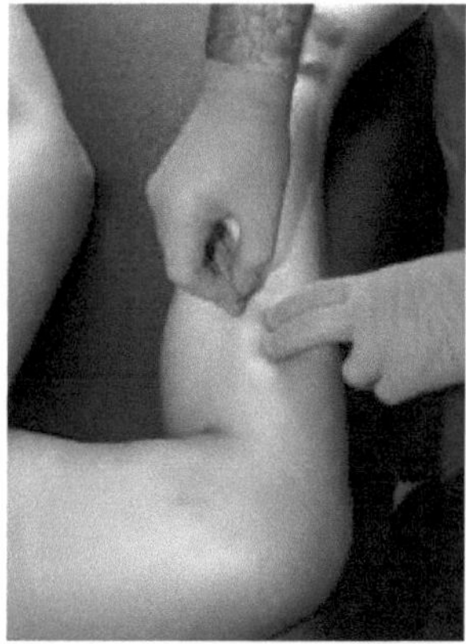

Figure 38. PS in PGM of the flexor digitorum longus (54).

5.4.6. Posterior tibial.

- PGMs in the posterior tibialis posterior muscle can be located at different heights along the muscle, and the referred pain pattern mainly affects the Achilles tendon, the back of the heel and the entire sole of the foot, occasionally extending to the toes and the central part of the calf. Patients with active PGMs in this muscle often experience pain when walking or running, especially on uneven surfaces, this being one of the main triggering mechanisms.

Improper footwear and hyperpronation of the foot also contribute to the activation of these points (101, 102).

- Dry needling: To perform dry needling in the posterior tibialis posterior muscle, a technique similar to that used in the flexor digitorum longus is recommended, with some variations in terms of needle depth and size. Direct palpation of the PGMs is impossible due to the depth of the muscle, so posterior pressure is performed through the calf muscles to locate the painful area. The needle is introduced from the medial aspect of the tibia in an anterolateral direction, making sure to keep it close to the tibia as a reference. In less recommended cases, there is an alternative technique in which the needle is inserted from the anterior aspect of the leg in an anteroposterior direction, passing through the tibialis anterior muscle and the interosseous membrane. However, this technique is less effective from a therapeutic point of view (101, 102).

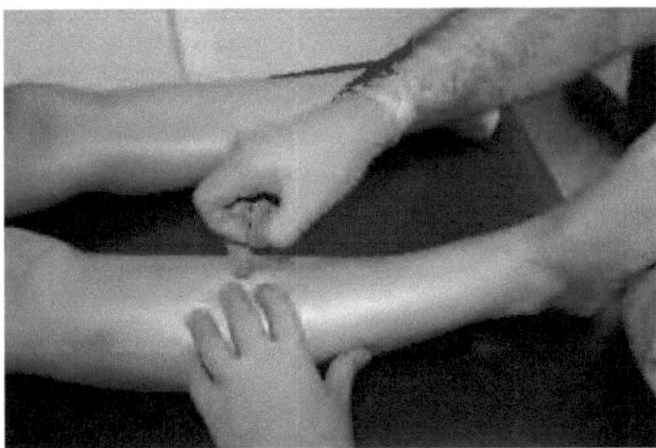

Figure 39. PS in PGM of the tibialis posterior from the anterior part of the leg (54).

- Dangers and precautions: In both techniques, there is a risk of affecting neurovascular structures such as the posterior tibial vessels and the tibial nerve. There may also be a risk of damaging the deep peroneal nerve if the needle is inserted too deeply and passes through the interosseous membrane. To minimize these risks, the needle should be kept as close to the tibia as possible (101, 102).

5.4.7. Flexor hallucis longus.

- PGMs in the flexor hallucis longus refer pain primarily to the plantar surface of the big toe and the head of the first metatarsal. The pain is usually related to walking and running, especially over uneven surfaces. These PGMs may also be responsible for muscle cramping and, in some cases, aggravate hallux valgus (bunion) by accentuating the valgus of the metatarsophalangeal joint (103, 104).
- Dry needling: To perform dry needling on the flexor hallucis longus, the patient should be placed in prone position with the foot outside the table. The physical therapist stands at the patient's feet and looks for the most sensitive point by deep flat palpation, in the direction of the posterior surface of the fibula, at or just above and below the junction of its middle and distal thirds. Once the hyperalgesic area is located, a 0.30 mm x 40 mm needle (or longer, depending on the thickness of the calf) is inserted, directed toward the fibula anteriorly and slightly laterally. Although not mandatory, it is recommended to make contact with the fibula to confirm correct depth and direction of the needle during exploration and treatment of the PGM (103, 104).

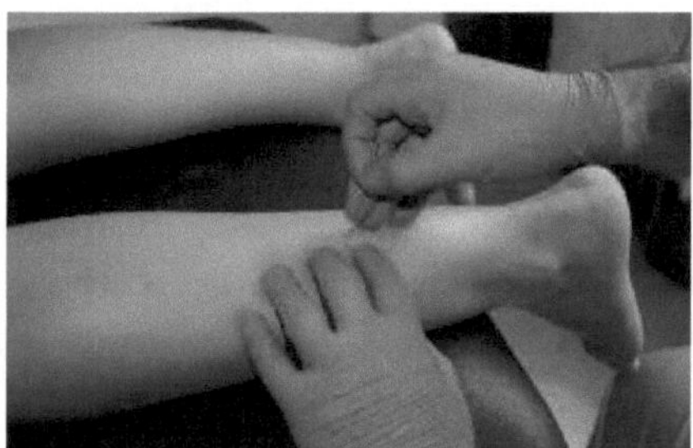

Figure 40. PS in PGM of the flexor hallucis longus (54).

- Hazards and precautions: The peroneal artery and veins are partially covered by the flexor hallucis longus muscle, which increases the risk of crossing these vascular structures during puncture. To minimize this risk, it is recommended to direct the needle slightly more laterally and avoid the most medial part of the fibula. If the patient experiences a prick or burning sensation before contacting the bone, this is a warning sign that the needle may be close to the vessels, requiring adjustment of the needle direction and application of adequate hemostatic pressure after the procedure (103, 104).

5.4.8. Anterior tibial.

- Tibialis anterior PGMs report pain primarily in the area where the tendon crosses the anteromedial aspect of the ankle and toward the big toe. Occasionally, pain radiates to the shin and anteromedial surface of the foot. In some cases, pain may be present at the proximal insertion of the muscle, at the lateral condyle of the tibia, without it being clear whether this is referred pain or a PGM in that area (103, 104).
- The patient with tibialis anterior MMPs may experience ankle weakness, resulting in frequent stumbling. Despite the overload that this muscle may experience, it is rare that nocturnal pain is reported due to these PGMs (103, 104).
- Activation mechanisms: Direct activation mechanisms of tibialis anterior PGMs include acute overloads, such as overstretching during forced plantar flexion or eccentric overload from tripping. Chronic overload from walking or running uphill, or even playing the bass drum on a drum kit, can also trigger PGMs in this muscle. However, shortening of antagonist muscles in the calf appears to be a frequent cause for the activation and persistence of these PGMs, making it essential to treat these antagonists (103, 104).
- Dry needling: The patient is placed in the supine position, while the physical therapist sits on the side to be treated. The PGM is located by flat palpation, and is crossed with a 0.25 mm x 40 mm needle directed medially until it contacts the tibia, which serves as a reference. The PGMs in this muscle are usually found superficially, in the peripheral location of the motor plates (103, 104).

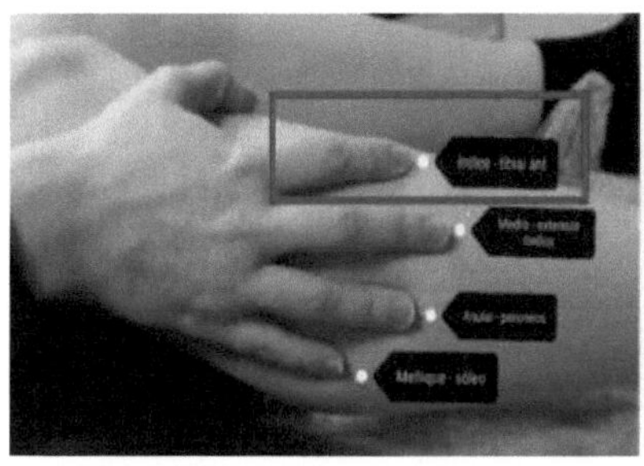

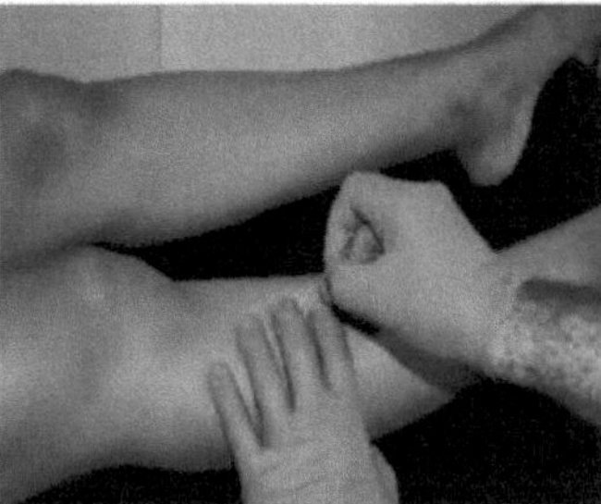

Figure 41. Reference and PS in PGM of the tibialis anterior (54).

- Dangers and precautions: The neurovascular bundle (anterior tibial artery and vein, and the deep peroneal nerve) runs just posterior to the tibialis anterior. To avoid damaging these structures, it is crucial to direct the needle medial to the tibia. There is a risk of developing anterior compartment syndrome from excessive bleeding, especially in patients with coagulopathies or taking anticoagulants. In these cases, in addition to considering the contraindication of dry needling, it is advisable to use thin needles, limit the use of aggressive techniques (such as multiple insertions), and be careful with ischemia during treatment and subsequent hemostasis (103, 104).

5.4.9. Peroneus longus and brevis.

- PGMs of the peroneus longus and peroneus brevis muscles project pain in the region of the lateral malleolus (both above, behind and below it) and along the lateral aspect of the foot. Peroneus longus PGMs may also refer pain along the lateral aspect of the leg.
- Symptoms and trigger mechanisms: Patients with PGMs in these muscles often present with ankle weakness and a tendency for sprains and strains, or even fractures. These injuries can lead to immobilization, which contributes to the perpetuation of MMPs. The two main mechanisms of PGM activation in the peroneals are (103, 104):
  - Acute eccentric overload: caused by a forced ankle inversion mechanism.

- Chronic overload: the result of static or dynamic imbalances of the foot, such as hyperpronation.

- Peroneal muscle PGMs are responsible for persistent pain in the lateral malleolus after sprains or fractures, and their treatment can improve concurrent instability and facilitate proprioceptive re-education. In addition, foot imbalances, such as flat feet, may activate or perpetuate peroneal PGMs, suggesting the need for podiatric evaluation to correct these problems with insoles. The possibility that peroneus longus PGMs may entrap the common peroneal nerve has also been described, which can lead to weakness in the muscles of the anterior and lateral compartments of the leg, and loss of sensation in the dorsum of the foot (103, 104).
- Dry needling: Dry needling of both peroneal muscles is performed in a similar manner, with variations due to their anatomical location. To locate the PGMs, flat palpation is used against the underlying fibula, and a 0.25 mm x 40 mm needle is inserted lateromedially toward the bone. The best position to perform the puncture is in contralateral decubitus, with the hip and knee flexed at about 90 degrees, which facilitates needle manipulation by the physical therapist (103, 104).

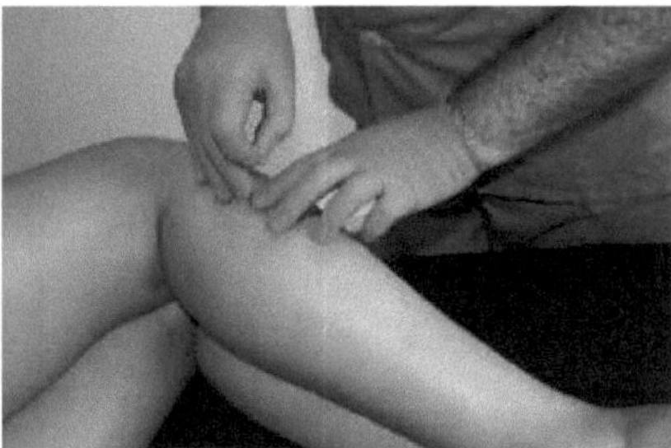

Figure 41. Peroneus longus (54).

- Dangers and precautions: In the proximal third of the peroneus longus muscle, there is a risk of accidental puncture of the common peroneal nerve, which passes under the muscle at that level. When puncturing the peroneus brevis muscle, a too anterior direction of the needle should be avoided in order not to injure the superficial peroneal nerve, which runs between the peroneus brevis and third peroneal muscles (103, 104).

5.4.10. Third peroneal.

- The referred pain pattern of myofascial trigger points (MTPs) of the third peroneal muscle projects primarily to the anterolateral aspect of the ankle and sometimes to the lateral surface of the heel. MTPs in this muscle may also contribute to a sensation of weakness in the ankle, similar to that caused by MTPs in the other two peroneals (long and short) (103, 104).
- Activation mechanisms: The third peroneus shares some activation mechanisms with the peroneus longus and peroneus brevis. However, its PGMs can be activated directly due to overloads or overstretching produced by forced inversion maneuvers combined with plantar flexion of the ankle, as occurs in activities such as hiking and certain sports that involve repetitive ankle movements in that position (103, 104).
- Dry needling: Identification of tight bands and elicitation of local twitch responses (REL) in this muscle is difficult by palpation. To locate the PGMs, the patient is placed in the supine position and dorsal flexion of the ankle combined with eversion and extension of the toes is requested. This allows visualization or palpation of the muscle tendon. Subsequently, hyperalgesia is sought in the anterolateral area of the distal third of the leg, pressing towards the fibula. Once the PGM is identified, a 0.25 mm x 40 mm needle is inserted in an anteroposterior direction with a slight lateral bias, seeking contact with the fibula to confirm the correct location (103, 104).

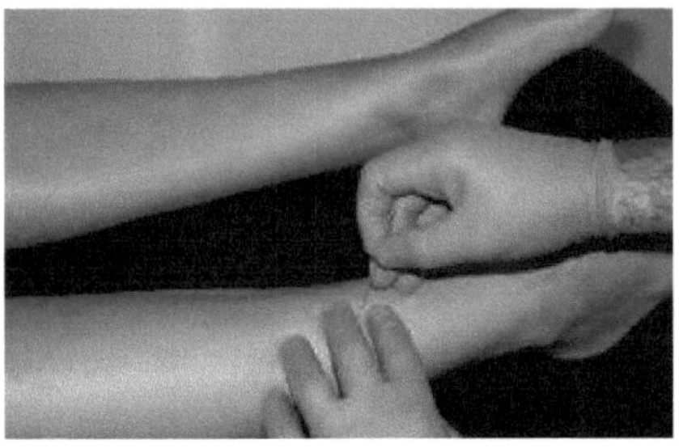

Figure 42. Third peroneal (54).

- Dangers and precautions: There is a risk of accidental puncture of the superficial peroneal nerve, which runs between the third peroneal and the peroneus brevis. To avoid this, it is important not to direct the needle excessively laterally, as this increases the possibility of contacting the nerve. Care should be taken to ensure that the needle reaches the fibula to minimize this risk (103, 104).

5.4.11. Long extensor of the fingers.

- Extensor digitorum longus PGMs can be found at different heights in the leg and often project their pain down the dorsum of the foot and toes, sometimes reaching almost halfway up the leg above and to the tips of the second to fourth toes below. Associated painful symptoms may include a feeling of weakness in ankle dorsiflexion, which affects control of foot drop during gait. This weakness can be especially intense if the PGMs cause entrapment of the deep peroneal nerve, which can cause neuroapraxia, affecting the strength of the muscles it innervates, such as the tibialis anterior, extensor digitorum longus, extensor hallucis longus and third peroneus. In many cases, the effects of this neuroapraxia can disappear within minutes after treatment of the extensor digitorum longus PGMs (101, 102, 103, 104).
- The most common mechanisms of PGM activation in extensor digitorum longus include (101, 102, 103, 104):
  - Acute overloads: caused by trips, falls, ankle sprains with plantar flexion, toe flexion and inversion.

- Chronic overloads: which can result from sustained shortening or stretching of the muscle. Examples include prolonged use of car pedals, wearing high heels, or certain sitting habits with the feet flexed under the chair.
- In addition, indirect mechanisms, such as lumbar radiculopathy or the presence of latent PGMs in the plantar flexor muscles, may be important factors in the development and perpetuation of PGMs in this muscle.

- Clinical (101, 102, 103, 104):
  - Pain: in the dorsum of the foot and toes.
  - Weakness: in ankle dorsiflexion.
  - Cramps: nocturnal muscle cramps.
  - Related muscles: plantar flexors.
- The dry needling technique for extensor digitorum longus is performed as follows (101, 102, 103, 104):
  - Patient position: Supine decubitus, with the physical therapist seated on the side to be treated.
  - PGM localization: Using flat palpation, the PGM is located and fixed by forking it between two fingers.
  - Needle insertion: A 0.25 mm x 40 mm needle is inserted with an anteroposterior trajectory, slightly adjusting the lateral, neutral or, very rarely, medial angle, depending on the location of the PGM. The needle should be directed towards the fibula bone.

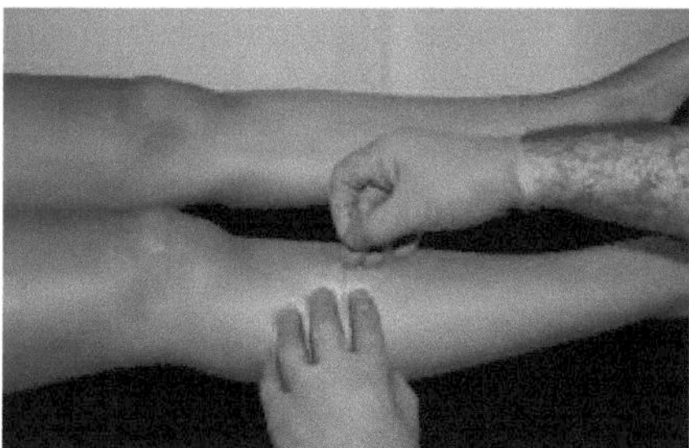

Figure 43. Long extensor of the fingers (54).

- Dangers and precautions: The deep peroneal nerve is located below the proximal part of the extensor digitorum longus, lying between this muscle and the tibialis anterior in the lower leg. Therefore, it is essential to direct the needle toward the fibula to minimize, but not eliminate, the risk of unwanted contact with the nerve. If the needle is directed excessively lateral and superficial, it could break with the superficial peroneal nerve, which runs lateral to the extensor digitorum longus. The variability in the location of the veins and the anterior tibial artery in relation to the fibula also advises seeking the fibula as a safer option during the procedure (101, 102, 103, 104).

5.4.12. Long extensor of the big toe.

- Myofascial trigger points (MTrPs) of the extensor hallucis longus present a referred pain pattern that mainly occupies the dorsum of the first metatarsal and may extend proximally to the location of the MTrP and distally to the tip of the big toe. A Spanish physiotherapist has documented a different pain pattern in patients who underwent a forced ankle inversion mechanism, which projects to the anterior fascicle of the deltoid ligament. In a series of 20 patients, treatment of this PGM has been successful in improving the often insidious pain of this ligament, which is a common sequela of external ankle sprains. In addition to pain, PGMs of the extensor hallucis longus can cause a sensation of weakness on ankle dorsiflexion, although they are not a cause of nerve entrapment. Similar to extensor digitorum longus, these PGMs may be associated with cramping, either at night or during sports activities such as swimming (105, 106).
- The mechanisms of PGM activation and perpetuation in the extensor hallucis longus are largely similar to those in the extensor digitorum longus. These include (105, 106):
    - Acute overloads: These can be caused by activities that involve excessive dorsiflexion, such as tripping or ankle sprains.

- Chronic overloads: Prolonged use of inappropriate footwear or postural habits that keep the muscle under tension can contribute to the development of MMPs.

- Clinical (105, 106):
    - Pain: In the dorsum of the first metatarsal.
    - Weakness: In ankle dorsiflexion.
- The dry needling (DOT) technique for the extensor pollicis longus toe PGMs is similar to that of the extensor digitorum longus, except for its more caudal and slightly more medial location (105, 106):
    - Patient position: Supine decubitus.
    - PGM localization: Palpation to identify the PGM in the muscle.
    - Needle insertion: A 0.25 mm x 40 mm needle is used. The needle should be directed towards the fibula with a slight lateral angulation, contacting the bone as a reference to determine the depth and probing slightly medial to the bone, thus exploring the most medial part of the muscle that inserts into the interosseous membrane.

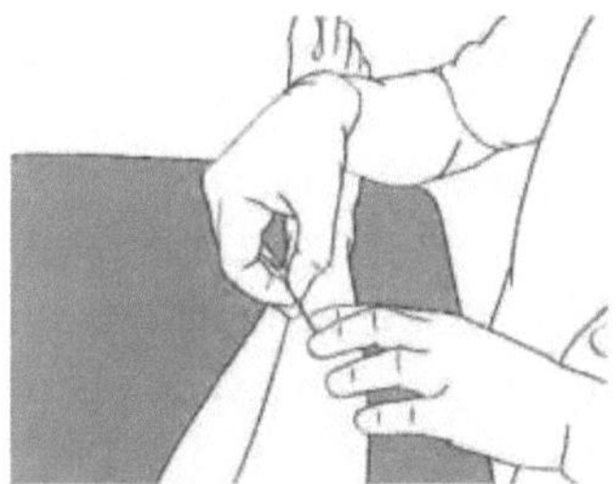
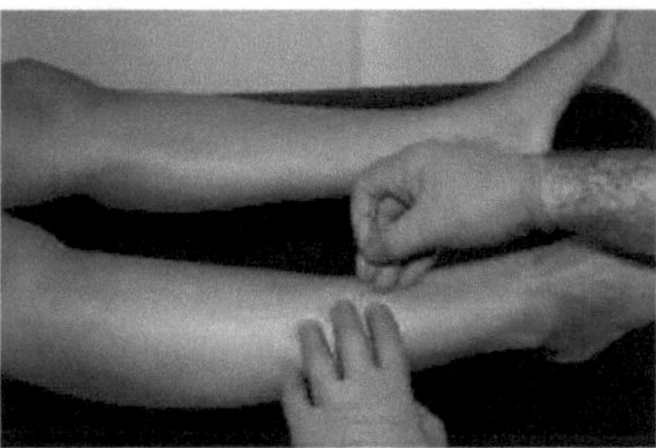

Figure 43. Long extensor of the great toe (53, 54).

- Hazards and Precautions: In the proximal part of the extensor hallucis longus, the neurovascular bundle formed by the anterior tibial vessels and the deep peroneal nerve is located lateral to the tendon of the muscle, in the superior and fleshy part, where the PGMs are commonly found. This neurovascular bundle is medial to the muscle, between the muscle and the tibialis anterior. For this reason, PS of the PGMs of the extensor hallucis longus carries the risk of affecting these structures. To minimize the risk we should avoid inserting the needle too close to the medial border of the muscle and direct the needle with a lateral bias towards the fibula (105, 106).

5.4.13. Flexor digitorum brevis and extensor digitorum brevis of the great toe.

- Myofascial trigger points (MTrPs) of the extensor digitorum brevis and extensor hallucis brevis muscles produce a pattern of referred pain that spreads across the mid-dorsum of the foot and may encompass the entire metatarsal region. This pain is often felt as diffuse discomfort in the area, which can hinder the mobility of the foot and limit the ability to perform daily activities (105, 106).
- The mechanisms of PGM activation in these muscles can be direct or a combination of direct and indirect. Some of the main factors that may contribute to their activation are described below (105, 106):
  - Excessive compression: Prolonged use of tight shoes or the habit of leaning on the foot can cause an activation and perpetuation of the PGMs in the short extensors.
  - Overloading and overstretching: Eccentric overloading due to sprains that force ankle inversion, associated with plantar flexion, can cause activation of the PGMs in both the short extensors and extensor digitorum longus. This overload could also cause dislocations or subluxations in the metatarsophalangeal joints, resulting in persistent activation of the PGMs.
  - Confusing diagnosis: This situation can lead to misdiagnosis, such as "foot sprain", where the patient feels pain in the dorsum of the foot without the typical signs of an external ankle sprain. Frequently, this discomfort is attributed to injuries of the medial ankle ligaments, but it could be related to activation of the extensor pollicis brevis PGMs. Activation of the extensor digitorum longus PGMs during the same trauma may also be an

indirect mechanism that perpetuates short extensor PGM activity.

- Clinical: Pain in the medial part of the dorsum of the foot. Related muscles extensor digitorum longus (105, 106).
- The dry needling technique to treat PGMs in the short extensors is as follows: Supine. The tense band and the PGM are identified by flat palpation. A 0.16 mm x 25 mm needle is inserted perpendicular to the skin in the direction of the PGM until it contacts the underlying bone (105, 106).

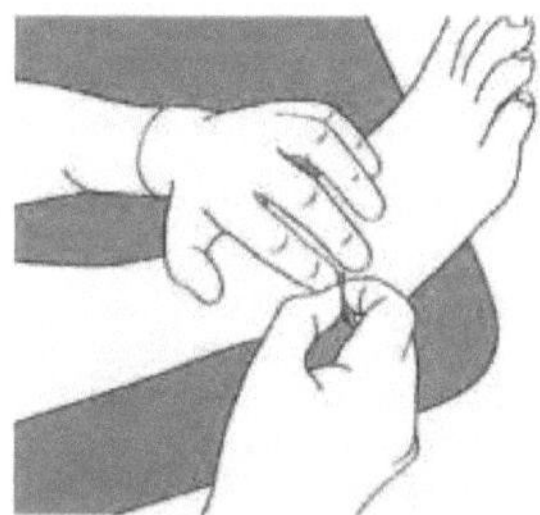
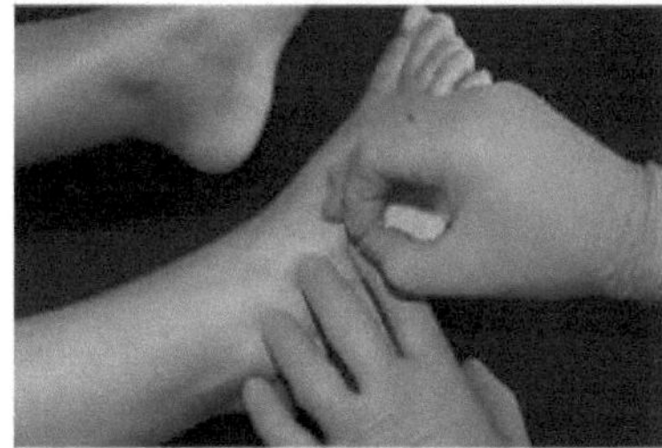

Figure 44. Extensor digitorum brevis of the great toe (53, 54).

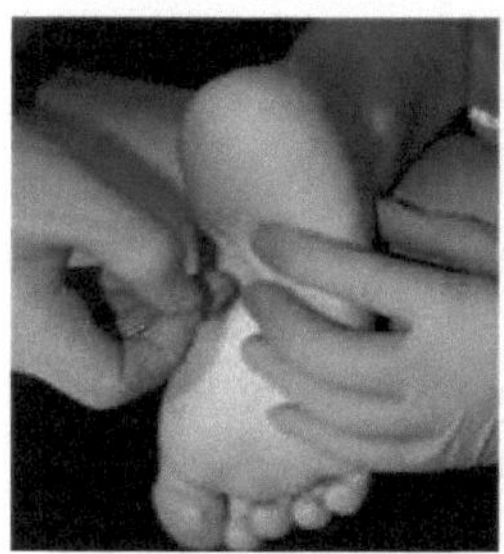
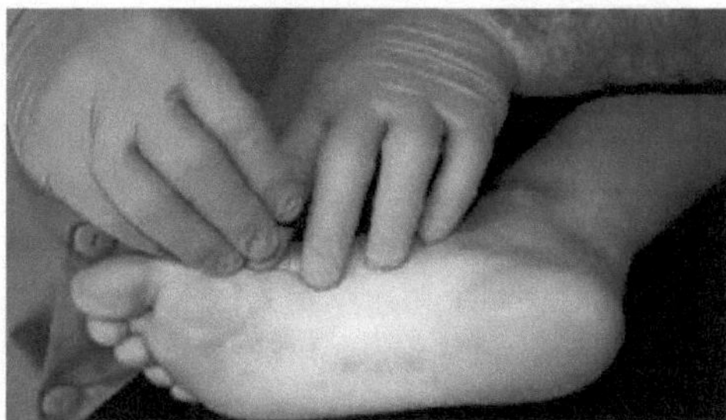

Figure 45. Flexor digitorum brevis of the great toe (53, 54).

- Hazards and precautions: It is essential to be aware of the following risks when performing dry needling in this area (105, 106):
    - Deep peroneal nerve and dorsal vessels of the foot: These structures run along the medial border of the extensor digitorum brevis muscle. Therefore, when performing the puncture, medial bias of the needle should be avoided.

- Pre-inspection: It is recommended to perform a visual inspection of the area before inserting the needle to identify cutaneous blood vessels or branches of the intermediate dorsal cutaneous nerve, which comes from the superficial peroneal nerve. This helps to avoid accidental punctures of these structures and minimize risks during the procedure.

5.4.14. Big toe abductor.

- Myofascial trigger points (MTrPs) of the abductor hallucis muscle are associated with a referred pain pattern that is primarily located at the medial border of the heel. This pain may extend to the posterior and medial aspect of the midfoot, as well as to the inner plantar arch. This pain pattern can be significant in the evaluation of patients with foot pain (107, 108).
- The PGMs of the abductor hallucis muscle can be activated by several factors (107, 108):
  - Wearing tight shoes: Constant pressure from shoes that do not fit properly can cause PGM activation.
  - Trauma: Injuries to the foot, including fractures, can contribute to PGM activation in this muscle.
  - Chronic overloads: Conditions such as flat feet or hypopronation can generate overloads that activate the PGMs. This is common in foot structures of particular morphology, which can lead to improper foot mechanics.
  - Plantar fasciitis: Active PGMs are frequently found in patients diagnosed with plantar fasciitis, and treatment of these trigger points often contributes to the patient's clinical improvement.
- Clinical: Pain in the medial border of the heel and in the medial part of the midfoot (107, 108).
- Related muscles: It could be associated with other intrinsic muscles of the foot, such as the flexors and extensors of the toes (107, 108).
- The dry needling technique for treating PGMs in the abductor hallucis muscle is as follows (107, 108):

- Patient position: The patient may be in homolateral decubitus or supine decubitus with the hip in external rotation. In both cases, the knee should be slightly flexed to facilitate access to the medial aspect of the foot.
- Physiotherapist access: The physiotherapist sits next to the patient at knee level. The patient's knee should be blocked by the physical therapist's arm and armpit to prevent sudden movements of the foot during the procedure, thus ensuring comfortable access to the foot.
- PGM localization: Flat palpation is used to locate the PGM and a 0.16 mm x 25 mm needle is inserted in the direction of the PGM, aiming to reach the underlying bone. In this position, the patient's big toe is free to move, allowing local responses (REL) to be perceived, such as movement of the toe towards abduction or flexion.

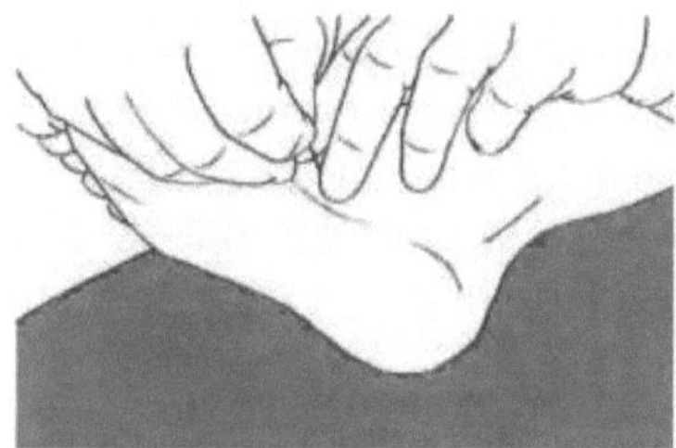
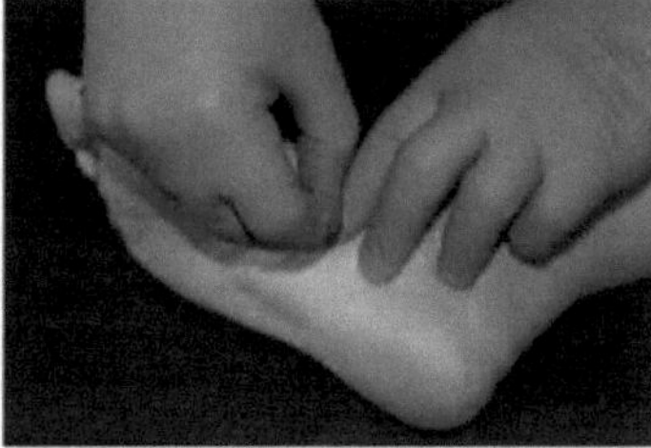

Figure 46. Big toe abductor (53, 54).

- Dangers and precautions: It is essential to follow certain precautions when performing dry needling in this area to avoid complications. In the proximal third of the muscle, the neurovascular bundle formed by the posterior tibial vessels and the medial and lateral plantar nerves lies just below the muscle. Therefore, care should be taken when inserting the needle in this area to avoid injury. By following these guidelines, dry needling can be performed effectively and safely, relieving the pain associated with PGMs of the abductor hallucis muscle and improving foot function (107, 108).

5.4.15. Abductor of the fifth finger.

- Myofascial trigger points (MTrPs) of the fifth toe abductor muscle can be found in various locations along this muscle. They generally project their referred pain to the plantar aspect of the fifth metatarsal head and can extend both distally and, especially, proximally, including parts of the metatarsal itself (107, 108).
- PGMs in the fifth finger abductor muscle can be activated by several factors, including (107, 108):
  - Tight Footwear: Similar to other intrinsic foot muscles, wearing shoes that do not fit properly can be both a trigger and perpetuator of PGMs in this muscle.
  - Hyperpronation of the foot: This type of foot deformity, which causes an excessive load on the muscles and ligaments, can be a determining factor for the appearance of PGM in the fifth toe abductor.
- Clinical: Localized pain in the plantar aspect of the fifth metatarsal head, often radiating towards the metatarsal and causing discomfort during activities involving foot loading (107, 108).
- Related muscles: Although the focus is on the fifth toe abductor, activation of other intrinsic foot muscles may also be related (107, 108).
- The dry needling technique for PGMs of the fifth finger abductor muscle is performed as follows (107, 108):
  - Patient position: The patient should be positioned in contralateral decubitus, with the affected lower limb behind the healthy one. This allows the medial edge of the affected foot to rest on the stretcher, leaving the lateral edge accessible for treatment.
  - Physiotherapist access: The physiotherapist is positioned in a manner similar to the technique used in abductor hallucis puncture.
  - PGM location and puncture: The PGMs can be palpated by pressing the muscle against the fifth metatarsal using a pincer palpation technique. A 0.16 mm x 25 mm needle is inserted

medial and dorsal to the underlying bone. In this position, the fifth toe is free to move, allowing observation of local responses (REL), such as abduction and flexion movements of the toe during the puncture.

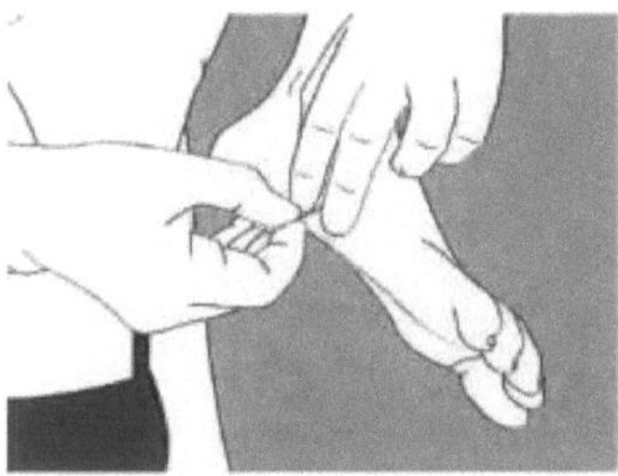
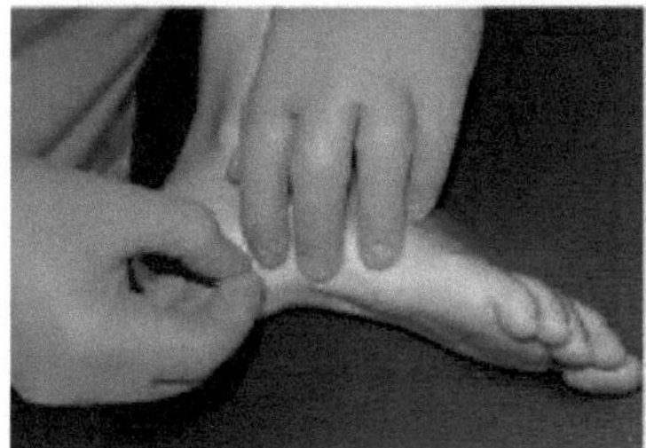

Figure 47. Abductor of the fifth finger (53, 54).

- Hazards and precautions When performing dry needling, certain precautions should be taken to avoid complications: The close relationship between the lateral plantar vessels and nerves and the inferomedial border of the fifth toe abductor muscle suggests that the needle should be inserted in a lateromedial direction, dorsally inclined, to minimize the risk of accidental puncture of these structures (107, 108).

5.4.16. Flexor digitorum brevis.

- Myofascial trigger points (MTrPs) of the flexor digitorum brevis muscle generate referred pain that projects mainly to the plantar area, specifically to the heads of the second through fourth metatarsals, and can sometimes extend to the head of the fifth metatarsal (109).
- PGMs in this muscle can be activated by several factors, among which the most important are (109):
  - Physical activities: walking on tiptoe, wearing high heels, dancing, and walking on uneven or unstable surfaces can trigger or perpetuate PGM activity in the flexor digitorum brevis.
  - Biomechanical alterations: Problems such as flat feet or hyperpronation can also contribute to the presence and

persistence of PGMs in this muscle. In some cases, consultation with a podiatrist may be necessary to create a corrective insole, although this may initially aggravate symptoms until the PGMs in the involved muscles are treated.
    - Relationship with other muscles: It is important to mention the connection between the PGMs of the flexor digitorum brevis and those of the calf muscles, such as the gastrocnemius, soleus, flexor digitorum longus and tibialis posterior, which can also project pain to the sole of the foot.
- Clinical: Patients usually experience metatarsalgia, i.e. pain in the forefoot, specifically in the metatarsal heads (109).
- Related muscles: In addition to the flexor digitorum brevis, it is related to the gastrocnemius, soleus, flexor digitorum longus and tibialis posterior muscles (109).
- The dry needling technique for PGMs of the flexor digitorum brevis muscle is performed as follows (109):
    - Patient position: The patient may be supine or prone.
    - PGM localization: Flat palpation is used to explore the sole of the foot for areas of focal pressure tenderness. It can be difficult to differentiate whether the tenderness is due to PGMs of the flexor digitorum brevis, plantar aponeurosis problems, plantar square muscle, or a combination of these factors.
    - Assessment test: A useful test is to maintain painful pressure on the hyperalgesic area and then passively extend the metatarsophalangeal joints of the toes. If this increases pain, it suggests a problem in the plantar aponeurosis. If, on the other hand, stretching the aponeurosis reduces the pain, it is likely that the PGMs of the flexor digitorum brevis or plantar quadratus are responsible.
    - Performance of the puncture: Dry needling is usually effective for plantar pain, regardless of the specific cause. It is recommended to use a 0.25 mm x 40 mm needle, directing it towards the tender area in a plantar to dorsal direction, until

reaching the bone as a reference, ensuring that the involved structures have been crossed.

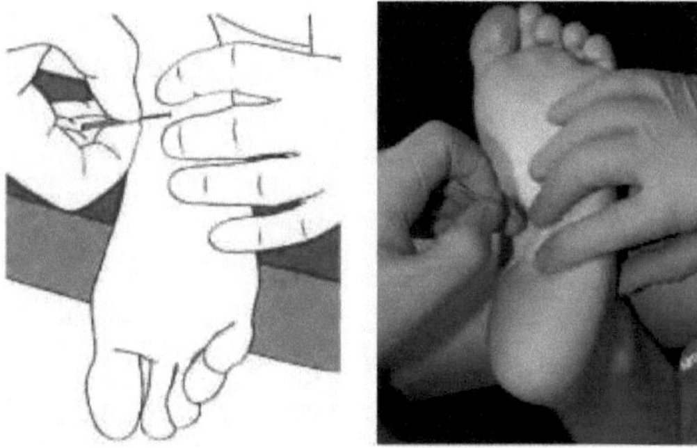

Figure 48. Flexor digitorum brevis (53, 54).

- Dangers and precautions: It is essential to be aware of the proximity of the lateral plantar vessels and nerves and, to a lesser extent, the medial plantar nerve, which run between the flexor digitorum brevis and the plantar quadratus muscle. Correct identification and treatment of the PGMs of the flexor digitorum brevis muscle through dry needling can provide significant pain relief and improve foot function (109).

5.4.17. Plantar square.

- Myofascial trigger points (MTPs) of the plantar square muscle often project their referred pain to the entire plantar surface of the heel. Identification and palpation of these PGMs can be challenging, as their location is often obscured by (110).
  - Soft tissues: Skin and plantar aponeurosis.
  - Adjacent muscles: Such as the flexor digitorum brevis (PGM on the medial head) and abductor digitorum cinque (PGM on the lateral), which may have their own active PGMs.
- The mechanisms that activate and perpetuate the PGMs of the plantar square muscle are similar to those of the flexor digitorum brevis and may include (110):

- Physical activities: Certain activities that require prolonged or improper use of the foot, such as walking or running on hard or unstable surfaces.
- Biomechanical alterations: Structural problems of the foot such as hyperpronation or lack of adequate support, which can contribute to plantar pain.
- Relationship with other muscles: The PGMs of the plantar square are related to other calf muscles, such as the gastrocnemius, soleus, tibialis posterior, and flexor digitorum longus, as well as the abductor hallucis. Tension or dysfunction in these muscles can affect the function of the plantar quadratus and vice versa.

- Clinical: Patients may experience pain throughout the sole of the foot, particularly in the heel, which may affect their ability to perform daily activities (110).
- Related muscles: In addition to the quadratus plantaris, the gastrocnemius, soleus, posterior tibialis, flexor digitorum longus and abductor hallucis (110) are involved.
- The recommended dry needling technique for treating plantar square PGMs is described as follows (110):
  - Palpation: Follow the previous instructions to locate the PGMs of the flexor digitorum brevis, using flat palpation and exploring the sole of the foot for hypersensitive areas.
  - Puncture technique: There are two approaches to puncture:
  - The recommended technique involves inserting the needle in a plantar to dorsal direction until the underlying bone is reached, as described for the flexor digitorum brevis.
  - An alternative approach involves inserting the needle in a mediolateral direction, just below the bony plane, which may be more tolerable for the patient and with less risk of accidental puncture. However, some authors consider this technique to be less effective and should be reserved for patients with low pain.
- Hazards and precautions: The hazards and precautions during dry needling of the PGMs of the quadratus plantaris muscle are similar

to those described for the flexor digitorum brevis. It is crucial to consider the following (110):

- Proximity of neurovascular structures: The proximity of nerves and plantar vessels may increase the risk of injury during puncture, so asepsis and safety instructions should be strictly followed during the procedure.
- The identification and treatment of plantar square muscle PGMs through dry needling can significantly aid in the reduction of plantar pain and improve the quality of life of patients suffering from metatarsalgia or chronic foot pain.

5.4.18. Flexor digitorum brevis of the great toe.

- Myofascial trigger points (MTrPs) of the flexor hallucis brevis muscle are characterized by a pattern of referred pain that projects primarily to the plantar and medial surfaces of the first metatarsal head. Sometimes, the pain spills over into the entire big toe and part of the second toe. These PGMs may be responsible for symptoms such as cramps in the big toe. It has also been observed that they can cause altered sensation in the form of tingling or swelling in the distal part of the foot, especially when associated with the PGMs of the flexor digitorum brevis of the fifth toe and the adductor hallucis (111).
- The PGMs of the flexor hallucis brevis can be activated by a variety of factors, including (111).
    - Inappropriate footwear: Wearing shoes that are too tight or improperly designed can trigger the activation of these points.
    - Trauma: Fractures of the bones of the foot or any other type of trauma to the area may be responsible.
- Perpetuating factors (111).
    - Cooling of the foot.
    - Walking on uneven or unstable terrain.
    - Hyperpronation of the foot, which may be associated with biomechanical dysfunctions.

- In addition, the PGMs of other synergistic or related muscles that project pain to the sole of the forefoot, such as the tibialis posterior, flexor hallucis longus, abductor hallucis, flexor digitorum brevis, and interossei, may contribute to the activation and perpetuation of the PGMs of the flexor hallucis brevis.

- Clinical: Pain commonly presents on the plantar and medial surfaces of the first metatarsal head, which may influence normal foot function (111).
- Related Muscles: Muscles frequently associated with PGMs of the flexor hallucis brevis include: Posterior tibialis, flexor hallucis longus, abductor hallucis, flexor digitorum brevis, interossei (111).
- The dry needling technique for the PGMs of the flexor digitorum brevis of the great toe is performed as follows (111):
  - Patient positioning: The patient should be in lateral decubitus on the affected side.
  - Localization and palpation: The PGM is located by flat palpation and pressure is maintained.
  - Needle insertion: A 0.25 mm x 40 mm needle is used. The needle is inserted just below the first metatarsal bone, in a mediolateral direction. The depth of insertion will depend on whether it is desired to reach only the medial head or also the lateral head.
  - Confirmation of puncture: The appearance of abrupt plantar flexion movements in the metarso-phalangeal joint of the big toe is observed, which confirms the correct puncture of the PGM.

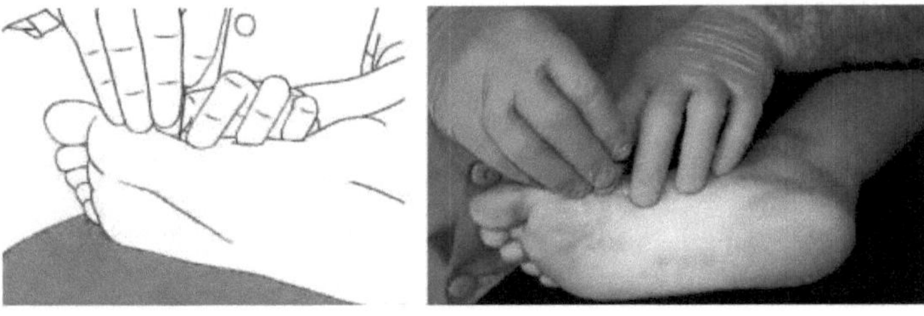

Figure 49. Flexor digitorum brevis and adductor hallucis (53, 54).

- Hazards and precautions (111):
  - Nerve puncture risk: Depending on the height at which the PGM is located, there is a possibility of the needle contacting the digital nerve proper or, more commonly, the common digital nerve, which is located near the plantar aspect of the medial head of the muscle. Therefore, the needle should be kept close to the bone and proper precautions should be followed.
  - Vascular risk: During the procedure, the needle could cross the plantar cutaneous venous arch or, rarely, the medial plantar artery. It is therefore essential to maintain adequate pressure during the puncture with the palpating hand and to perform good hemostasis immediately after the puncture.
  - Proper management of the PGMs of the flexor digitorum brevis muscle by dry needling may be an effective approach to relieve pain and improve foot function in patients with chronic plantar pain.

5.4.19. Adductor of the big toe.

- Myofascial trigger points (MTrPs) of the adductor hallucis muscle have a referred pain pattern that extends along the sole of the foot, specifically covering the area between the first and fourth metatarsal heads. In addition, like the PGMs of other muscles such as the flexor hallucis brevis or flexor digitorum brevis of the fifth toe, they can cause dysesthesia, which manifests as tingling sensations and swelling throughout the distal part of the foot (109, 110, 111).
- The mechanisms of PGM activation and perpetuation in the great toe adductor are similar to those of other intrinsic foot muscles. These may include (109, 110, 111):
  - Inappropriate footwear: Footwear that does not provide adequate support or is too tight.
  - Trauma: Injuries to the foot, including fractures or sprains.
  - Perpetuating factors: Hyperpronation, walking on uneven surfaces, cooling of the foot.

- Dry puncture (109, 110, 111):
  - Technique for the oblique head: The oblique head of the adductor hallucis muscle lies in the same plane as the flexor hallucis brevis, in contact with its lateral head. The dry needling technique for this head is similar to that described for the flexor hallucis brevis, but the needle insertion is deeper and lateral. With the patient in lateral decubitus, the big toe should be left free to allow its movement. The needle (0.25 mm x 40 mm) is inserted in a lateral direction, and the appearance of sudden movements of the big toe towards the second toe will confirm the correct puncture of the PGM.
  - Transverse Head Technique: The PGMs of the transverse head can be reached directly from the sole of the foot. However, due to skin sensitivity and hardness of the area, a more indirect approach from the dorsum of the forefoot is recommended. The patient should be in the supine position. Deep palpation is used to locate painful tenderness to pressure, looking for the PGM immediately proximal to the metatarsal heads. The needle (0.25 mm x 40 mm) is inserted from the dorsum of the foot, in the direction of the palpating toe, passing through the interosseous space to reach the identified MTP.
- Dangers and precautions: Although the caliber of these nerves is small and the risk of damage is low, recommendations should be followed to avoid complications (109, 110, 111):
  - For the oblique head: Watch for the digital nerve proper and the common digital nerve. Be mindful of the plantar cutaneous venous arch and medial plantar artery. Maintain good aseptic practices during the procedure.
  - For the transverse head: insertion of the needle into the interosseous space carries the risk of affecting the medial or lateral branches of the superficial peroneal nerve, the deep peroneal nerve and the common plantar digital nerves.

5.4.20. Dorsal and plantar interosseous.

- Myofascial trigger points (MTrPs) of the interosseous muscles of the foot, both dorsal and plantar (and probably also the lumbrical muscles), generate referred pain that manifests on the side of the toe where the tendon inserts. This pain may also include dorsal and plantar areas along the distal part of the corresponding metatarsal (109, 110, 111).
- Associated symptoms (109, 110, 111):
    - Paresthesias: The first dorsal interosseous may cause tingling sensations in the big toe, which may extend to the dorsum of the foot and the anteroinferior part of the leg. Kellgren documented that first dorsal interosseous pain may radiate to the lateral half of the foot and calf.
    - Finger Deformity: As a result of the shortening caused by PGMs, the patient may complain that one finger is unusually close to another, or that the tip of one finger does not rest properly on the ground, resulting in difficulty in properly flexing the interphalanges.
    - Hammertoe: PGM-induced weakness of the dorsal interosseous may contribute to hammertoe deformity.
- Mechanisms of activation and perpetuation: The mechanisms that activate and perpetuate PGMs in the interosseous muscles are common to those described above for other plantar muscles. These may include (109, 110, 111):
    - Mechanical overload: Activities that overload the interosseous muscles.
    - Inappropriate footwear: Footwear that does not provide adequate support or is too narrow.
    - Trauma: Injuries or impacts to the foot region.
- Dry needling: The patient should be in the supine position. The physical therapist is positioned appropriately and uses a bimanual flat palpation technique to identify the PGM. Once located, the PGM is fixed with the thumb on the dorsum of the foot and the index and middle fingers on the sole, using a modified clamp palpation. A 0.16 mm x 25 mm needle is recommended. The needle

is inserted from the dorsum of the foot in the direction of the toes located on the sole, applying significant dorsal pressure to allow the needle to reach the heads of the dorsal interosseous and, if necessary, the corresponding plantar interosseous. Probing with the needle in the lateral and medial directions may be required, and it is important that the patient's toes have freedom of movement. Shaking of either toe in the direction of abduction or adduction, provoked by local reactions (REL), will help to identify which interosseous (dorsal or plantar) harbored the PGM (109, 110, 111).

- Dangers and precautions: Dry needling of the interosseous muscles is low risk if proper recommendations are followed. Precautions include taking care with the medial and lateral branches of the superficial peroneal nerve, as well as the medial terminal branch of the deep peroneal nerve, the common plantar digital nerves, and the medial plantar nerve, depending on the space through which the needle is inserted (109, 110, 111).

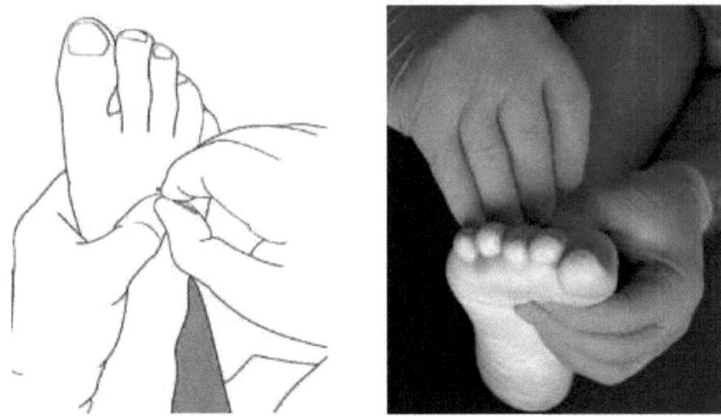

Figure 50. Dorsal and plantar interossei (53, 54).

5.4.21. Lateral capsuloligamentous structures of the ankle and foot.

- The treatment of non-myofascial trigger points (NMTPs) in the capsuloligamentous structures of the ankle and foot has been the subject of study for several decades. In particular, Dr. Travell and Dr. Audrie L. Bobb conducted significant research between 1941 and 1942 that addressed the effects of procaine and other injectable fluids in the treatment of trigger areas in fibrous connective tissues (1, 53).

- Travell's experiments: Dr. Travell described how to treat patients with acute ankle and knee sprains by identifying trigger areas in joint capsules, ligaments and tendons. This approach, focusing on targeted injections to specific pain points, proved effective, allowing patients to load on the injured joint and walk without pain after treatment (1, 53):
    - Procaine injection: Initially used, it was focused on specific trigger areas within the injured areas.
    - Isotonic Saline Solution: In some cases, it was used instead of procaine, proving to be equally effective.
    - Dry needling: This technique, which involves the direct puncture of trigger points with a needle, also showed good results, even without the administration of anesthetics.
- Research Results: Travell's findings were presented at a congress in 1947 and later published in 1952. In his article, several trigger areas related to external ankle sprains were highlighted, showing how referred pain extended to different regions of the ankle and foot (1, 53).
- Referred Pain: The pain associated with different PGNM can extend throughout the ankle and foot, affecting both the joint capsule and adjacent ligaments and tendons (1, 53).
- Importance of Location: It was observed that treating trigger points located under the fibula could be related to several capsuloligamentous structures and contribute to the treatment of pain in the medial collateral ligament area (1, 53).
- Clinical utility and future research: Despite the clinical utility observed in the treatment of PGNM in the ankle and other joints, there is a lack of rigorous documentation and studies on these practices. The use of modern techniques, such as ultrasound, could

provide a better characterization of trigger areas and their referred pain, as well as evidence on the actual efficacy of treatments, dosage, risks and contraindications (1, 53).

- Dry needle puncture: The use of 0.25 mm x 25 mm needles is recommended. They are inserted in the painful points located by palpation, following the indications previously described for dry needling of PGNM (1, 53).
- Hazards and precautions: Given the high probability of the needle contacting the joint capsule and potentially entering the joint, extreme asepsis and disinfection measures are crucial. Significant bruising at the puncture site may contraindicate the use of dry needling at some sites (1, 53).

Dry needling of PGNMs in the lateral capsuloligamentous structures of the ankle and foot may be a valuable technique in pain management. However, more research is needed to validate its efficacy and establish safe and effective protocols for its application.

Dry needling has established itself as an effective therapeutic technique in the treatment of myofascial trigger points (MTrPs) in the lower limbs, providing significant pain relief and improving muscle function. Its application on muscles such as the adductor, interosseous and foot flexors, as well as capsuloligamentous structures, demonstrates its versatility and efficacy. Clinical findings suggest that dry needling not only relieves localized pain, but can also positively influence referred pain perception and mobility of affected joints. Through direct stimulation of the PGMs, desensitization of hypersensitive areas is achieved, facilitating functional recovery and reducing disability.

However, it is essential to recognize the importance of adequate training of the physical therapist in the technique and the necessary precautions to minimize risks, such as possible injury to nerve or vascular structures. In addition, further research is required to deepen the understanding of the underlying mechanisms, as well as the validation of specific protocols and their effectiveness in different populations.

In conclusion, dry needling of the lower limbs represents a valuable tool in physical therapy, contributing to pain management and improvement of patients' quality of life. Its integration in a multidisciplinary treatment approach, along with other therapeutic modalities, can optimize clinical outcomes and enhance recovery in painful conditions of the locomotor system.

6. BIBLIOGRAPHICAL REFERENCES.

1. Simons, D.G., Travell, J.G., Simons, L.S. (2002). Myofascial pain and dysfunction: The trigger point manual. Upper half of the body, 2ed. Madrid: Editorial Médica Panamericana. ISBN: 9788479035754.
2. Dommerholt, J., Fernandez, C. (2018). Trigger Point Dry Needling: An Evidenced and Clinical-Based Approach. 2nd edition. Elselvier. ISBN: 978-0702074165.
3. American Physical Therapy Association (APTA). (2012). Physical therapists and the performance of dry needling. 1-141.
4. Baldry, P. (2005). Acupuncture, trigger points and musculoskeletal pain. 3rd ed. Churchill Livingstone. ISBN: 978-0443066443.
5. Hong, C.Z. (1994). Lidocaine injection versus dry needling to myofascial trigger points: The importance of the local twitch response. American Journal of Physical Medicine and Rehabilitation. 73(4): 256-263.
6. Cummings, T.M., White, A.R. (2001). Needling therapies in the management of myofascial trigger point pain: A systematic review. Archives of Physical Medicine and Rehabilitation. 82(7): 986-992.
7. Tough, E.A., White, A.R., Cummings, T.M., Richards, S.H., Campbell, J.L. (2009). Acupuncture and dry needling in the management of myofascial trigger point pain: A systematic review and meta-analysis of randomized controlled trials. European Journal of Pain. 13(1): 3-10.
8. Kietrys, D.M., Palombaro, K.M., Azzaretto, E. (2013). Effectiveness of dry needling for upper-quarter myofascial pain: A systematic review and meta-analysis. Journal of Orthopaedic and Sports Physical Therapy, 43(9): 620-634.
9. Peuker, E.T., White, A. (1999). Anatomy for the clinical practice of acupuncture. Clinical Anatomy. 12(3): 174-182.
10. Ernst, E., White, A.R. (2001). Prospective studies of the safety of acupuncture: A systematic review. American Journal of Medicine. 110(6): 481-485.

11. Cummings, T.M., Baldry, P. (2007). Regional myofascial pain: Diagnosis and management. Best Practice and Research Clinical Rheumatology. 21(2): 367-387.
12. Aldlyami, E., Kulkarni, A., Reed, M.R., Muller, S.D. (2010). Partington Latex-free gloves: safer for whom? J. Arthroplasty. 25: 27-30.
13. Mayoral, O. (2009). Trigger point dry needling: A simple technique for the treatment of myofascial pain. Fisioterapia. 31(3): 126-134.
14. Perez, L. (2020). Contraindications in dry needling therapy. Advances in physiotherapy. Springer. 245-260.
15. Morales, E. (2018). Assessment and risks in dry needling. In S. Fernandez (Ed.), Contemporary therapies in chronic pain. Editorial Médica. 115-130.
16. Rodriguez, A. (2021). Evaluation of the effectiveness and safety of dry needling in patients with muscle pain: a clinical study. Master's thesis, University of Barcelona.
17. Boyce, J.M., Pittet, D. (2002). Guideline for hand hygiene in health-care settings: Recommendations of the Healthcare Infection Control Practices Advisory Committee and the HICPAC/SHEA/APIC/IDSA Hand Hygiene Task Force. American Journal of Infection Control 30(8): S1-S46.
18. Health Service Executive (HSE). (2009). Standard precautions in health care. Health protection surveillance centre.
19. Yunus, M.B., and Mense, S. (2019). Myofascial pain syndrome and trigger points: clinical review and pathophysiology. Pain Medicine. 21(2): 179-190.
20. Cagnie, B., Dewitte, V., Barbe, T., Timmermans, F., Delrue, N. (2020). Needling therapies in the management of myofascial trigger points: A systematic review. American Journal of Physical Medicine and Rehabilitation. 99(4): 309-318.
21. Gattie, E., Cleland, J.A., Snodgrass, S.J. (2017). Dry needling for patients with musculoskeletal pain: A clinical commentary. International Journal of Sports Physical Therapy. 12(2): 227-236.
22. Kietrys, D. M., Palombaro, K. M., Azzaretto, E. (2019). Effectiveness of dry needling for upper-quarter myofascial pain: A systematic

review and meta-analysis. Journal of Orthopaedic and Sports Physical Therapy. 43(9): 620-634.

23. Shah, J. P., Thaker, N. (2018). Myofascial pain and nociceptive trigger points: Time to integrate dry needling with evidence-based medicine. The Journal of Orthopaedic and Sports Physical Therapy. 48(1): 3-9.
24. Melzack, R., Wall, P.D. (1965). Pain mechanisms: a new theory. Science, 150(3699): 971-979.
25. Dommerholt, J., Fernández-de-las-Peñas, C. (2013). Trigger Point Dry Needling: An Evidence and Clinical-Based Approach. Churchill Livingstone.
26. Shah, J.P., Gilliams, E.A. (2008). Uncovering the biochemical milieu of myofascial trigger points using in vivo microdialysis: An application of muscle pain concepts to myofascial pain syndrome. Journal of Bodywork and Movement Therapies. 12(4): 371-384.
27. Langevin, H.M., Yandow, J.A. (2002). Relationship of acupuncture points and meridians to connective tissue planes. The Anatomical Record. 269(6): 257-265.
28. Hidalgo, J., Torres, M., Mayoral, O., Sanchez, Z., Prieto, S. (2013). Infrared thermography for the detection of myofascial trigger points in patients with neck pain. Medical Physics. 40(7).
29. Dutton, M. (2018). Fundamentals of Musculoskeletal Assessment Techniques. 4th ed. New York: Elsevier.
30. Kettner, N., Ragnarsdottir, M. (2014). The Importance of Medical History and Physical Examination in the Clinical Setting. Journal of Physical Therapy Science. 26(4): 649-653.
31. Gillon, R. (2015). Informed Consent: A Guide for Healthcare Professionals. Journal of Medical Ethics. 41(5): 391-395.
32. Riazi, H., Dyer, C. B. (2016). Informed Consent: Ethical and Legal Considerations in Physical Therapy Practice. Physiotherapy Theory and Practice. 32(1): 37-46.
33. Groves, M. (2016). Documenting Informed Consent in Physical Therapy: An Ethical and Legal Imperative. Journal of Physical Therapy Education. 30(3): 15-22.

34. Schenck, K.L., Hall, R.M. (2018). Legal Considerations in Informed Consent for Physical Therapy. Journal of Legal Medicine. 39(3): 331-344.
35. McEwen, I.R., Pomeranz, B. (2015). Clinical Handbook of Physiotherapy. New York: Wiley.
36. Walker, J.A., Allen, S.S. (2017). Infection Control in Physical Therapy Practice. Journal of Physical Therapy Science. 29(9): 1665-1670.
37. Glover, J.E., Pomeranz, B. (2016). Patient Positioning and Ergonomics in Rehabilitation. Physical Therapy. 96(5): 617-626.
38. Sweeney, J., Murphy, A. (2019). Best Practices for Patient Positioning in Manual Therapy Techniques. Physiotherapy Theory and Practice. 35(2): 136-142.
39. Cummings, T.M., Cummings, T.J. (2015). Dry Needling: A Clinical Perspective. Journal of Manual and Manipulative Therapy. 23(3): 145-155.
40. Dommerholt, J. (2011). Myofascial Trigger Points: Pathophysiology and Evidence-Informed Diagnosis and Management. Journal of Manual and Manipulative Therapy. 19(3): 137-147.
41. Trevelyan, F.C., and Noyes, R.A. (2018). Post-Needling Care: Understanding the Role of Patient Education. Physical Therapy Reviews. 23(1): 22-31.
42. Alvarez, A. (2015). Dry needling: efficacy in the treatment of myofascial pain syndrome. International Journal of Medicine and Sciences of Physical Activity and Sport. 15(59): 245-258.
43. Sato, T., Rosen, J. (2020). Effects of dry needling on muscle pain: a systematic review. Physiotherapy Theory and Practice. 36(4): 428-441.
44. Ursini, T., Tontodonati, M. (2018). The role of inflammation in muscle regeneration. Current Opinion in Rheumatology. 30(1): 38-43.
45. Shah, J.P., Thaker, H. (2023). "Nonmyofascial Trigger Points: A Comprehensive Review." Journal of Pain Research. 16: 107-119.

46. Klein, M.J., et al. (2021). "Non-myo-fascial Trigger Points: An Underrecognized Cause of Pain." Journal of Bodywork and Movement Therapies. 25(4): 767-773.
47. Alvarez, D. J., Rockwell, P. G. (2022). "Understanding Non-Myo-Fascial Pain: A Review of Trigger Points and Related Conditions." Pain Medicine. 23(8): 1433-1442.
48. Meyer, M.F., et al. (2022). "Exploring the Mechanisms Behind Dry Needling in Non-myofascial Pain: An Evidence-Based Approach." Clinical Rehabilitation. 36(6): 760-771.
49. Tashjian, R.Z., et al. (2021). "Clinical Approaches to Nonmyofascial Trigger Points." Pain Physician. 24(2): 97-106.
50. Tough, E.A., White, A.R. (2022). "The Role of Dry Needling in Treating Non-Myo-fascial Pain." Current Pain and Headache Reports. 26(6): 455-462.
51. Dommerholt, J., Mayoral, O., Gröbli, C. (2006). Trigger point dry needling. journal of manual and manipulative therapy. 14(4): 70-87.
52. Chys, M., De Meulemeester, K., Murillo, C., De Greef, I. (2023). Clinical effectiveness of dry needling in patients with musculoskeletal pain-An Umbrella Review. Journal of Clinical Medicine. 12(3): 1205.
53. Mayoral, O., Salvat, I. (2021). Invasive physiotherapy of myofascial pain syndrome: trigger point dry needling manual. ISBN: 978-8491103950.
54. Dommerholt, J., Fernandez, C. (2013). Trigger Point Dry Needling: An Evidence and Clinical-Based Approach. Churchill Livingstone.
55. Kietrys, D.M., Palombaro, K.M., Azzaretto, E., Hubler, R., Schaller, B., Schlussel, J.M., et al. (2013). Effectiveness of dry needling for upper-quarter myofascial pain: A systematic review and meta-analysis. The Journal of Orthopaedic and Sports Physi-cal Therapy. 43(9): 620-34.
56. Boyles, R., Fowler, R., Ramsey, D., Burrows, E. (2015). Effectiveness of trigger point dry needling for multiple body regions: A systematic review. The Journal of Manual adn Manipulative Therapy. 23(5): 276-93.

57. Valera, F., Minaya, F. (2016). "Effects of dry needling on myofascial trigger points of the pectoralis major muscle in subjects with myofascial pain." Physiotherapy. 38(1): 24-32.
58. Cagnie, B., Dewitte, V., Barbe, T., Timmermans, F., Delrue, N., Meeus, M. (2013). "The Use of Dry Needling in the Management of Myofascial Trigger Points: A Pilot Study." Journal of Bodywork and Movement Therapies. 17(4): 424-429.
59. Fernandez, C., Dommerholt, J. (2014). "Dry Needling of the Pectoralis Major Muscle in Patients with Shoulder Pain: A Randomized Controlled Trial." Journal of Manual & Manipulative Therapy. 22(3): 155-162.
60. Calvo, C., et al. (2017). "Comparison of the Acute Effects of Dry Needling of Active Myofascial Trigger Points in the Pectoralis Major and Infraspinatus Muscles in Patients with Shoulder Pain." Journal of Manipulative and Physiological Therapeutics. 40(9): 616-623.
61. Simons, D. G. (2004). "Review of Effects of Dry Needling on Myofascial Trigger Points in the Upper Quarter Including the Pectoralis Major Muscle." Journal of Musculoskeletal Pain. 12(3-4): 123-134.
62. Perez, S., Olivan, B., Magallon, R., De la Torre, M., Gaspar, E., Romo, L., et al. (2010). Percutaneous electrical nerve stimulation versus dry needling: effectiveness in the treatment of chronic low back pain. J Musculoskelet Pain. 18(1): 23-30.
63. Furlan, A.D., Van Tulder, M., Cherkin, D., Tsukayama, H., Lao, L., Koas, B., et al. (2005). Acupuncture and dry-needling for low back pain: an updated systematic review within the framework of the cochrane collaboration. Spine. 30(8): 944-63.
64. Athanasakis, P., Nikodelis, T., Panoutsakopoulos, V, Mylonas, V. (2024). Acute effect of dry needling on trunk kinematics and balance of patients with non-specific low back pain.
65. Hu, H.T., Gao, H., Ma, R.J., Zhao, X.F., Tian, H.F., Li, L. (2018). Is dry needling effective for low back pain: a systematic review and meta-analysis according to PRISMA. Medicine. 97: e11225.

66. Fernandez, C., Dommerholt, J. (2014). Dry Needling of the Thoracic Multifidi Muscles in Patients with Chronic Thoracic Spine Pain: A Case Series. Journal of Bodywork and Movement Therapies. 18(1): 145-151.
67. Boyle, K.L., Olinick, J., Lewis, C. (2010). The Value of Blending Dry Needling with Chiropractic Spinal Manipulation for Patients with Chronic Thoracic Spine Pain. Journal of Chiropractic Medicine. 9(2): 79-86.
68. Liu, L., Huang, Q.M., Liu, Q.G., Thitham, N., Li, L.H., Ma, Y.T., Zhao, J.M. (2018). Evidence for dry needling in the treatment of myofascial trigger points associated with low back pain: a systematic review and meta-analysis. 99(1):144-152.e2.
69. Khan, I., Ahmad, A., Ahmed, A., Sadiq, S., Asim, H.M. (2021). Effects of dry needling on myofascial trigger points of the lower extremities. J. Pak. Med. Assoc. 71: 2596-2603.
70. Morihisa, R., Eskew, J., McNamara, A., Young, J. (2016). Dry needling in subjects with lower quarter muscle trigger points: a systematic review. Int. J. Sports Phys. Ther. 11 :1-14.
71. Meleger, A.L., Krivickas, L.S. (2007). Neck and back pain: musculoskeletal disorders. Neurol. Clin. 25: 419-438.
72. García, M., Peña, S., Martín, M. (2021). Effectiveness of dry needling on myofascial trigger points in athletes: systematic review. Andalusian Journal of Sports Medicine. 14(2): 66-74.
73. Dommerholt, J., Huijbregts, P. (2010). Myofascial Trigger Points: Pathophysiology and Evidence-Informed Diagnosis and Management. Jones & Bartlett Learning. ISBN: 978-0763779740.
74. Huguenin, L., Brukner, P.D., McCrory, P., Smith, P., Wajswelner, H., Bennell, K. (2005). Effect of dry needling of gluteal muscles on straight leg raise: a randomised, placebo controlled, double blind trial. Br J Sports Med. 39: 84-90.
75. Onik, G., Kasprzyk, T., Knapik, K., Wieczorek, K. (2020). Myofascial Trigger Points Therapy Modifies Thermal Map of Gluteal Region. BioMed Research International. 24.

76. Zarei, H., Bervis, S., Piroozi, S., Motealleh, A. (2019). Added value of gluteus medius and quadratus lumborum dry needling in improving knee pain and function in female athletes with patellofemoral pain: a randomized clinical trial. Archives of Physical Medicine and Rehabilitation. 101.
77. Reina, F., Dommerholt, J., Fernandez, C. (2017). Myofascial Trigger Points, Pain, and Dry Needling in the Iliotibial Band Syndrome. Pain Medicine. 18(3): 550-555.
78. Rodríguez, J., González, B., De la casa, M., Salín, L., Martín, P. (2016). Efficacy of dry needling and other invasive techniques in piriformis syndrome. International Journal of Sport Science Research. 12(3): 131-145.
79. Boyajian, L.A., McClain, R.L., Coleman, M.K., Thomas, P.P. (2008). Diagnosis and management of piriformis syndrome: An osteopathic approach. Journal of the American Osteopathic Association. 108(11): 657-664.
80. Mayoral, O., Salvat, I., Hernández, P. (2013). Efficacy of deep dry needling on myofascial trigger points of the rectus abdominis muscle in patients with chronic low back pain. International Journal of Sport Science Research. 9(32): 297-306.
81. Tesch, P. A., & Lindberg, F. (2014). Effects of dry needling on muscle activation and pain in the rectus abdominis muscle during exercise. International Journal of Sports Physical Therapy. 9(6): 803-809.
82. Dommerholt, J. (2010). Dry needling of the obliquus internus and obliquus externus abdominis muscles. Journal of Bodywork and Movement Therapies, 14(4): 394-398.
83. Ríos Bautista, A., & Domínguez Molina, S. (2012). Deep dry needling in the treatment of abdominal myofascial syndrome. Fisioterapia. 34(5): 236-244.
84. Mayoral, O., Salvat, I., Martín, M.T., Martín, A.M., Calvo, M. (2012). Efficacy of deep dry needling on myofascial trigger points of the sartorius muscle in patients with chronic pain. Journal of Physical Therapy. 35(2): 120-125.

85. Zarrin, M., Nakhosin, N., Naghdi, S., Hasson, S., Forogh, B., Rezaee, M. (2023). Dry Needling for Arthrogenic Muscle Inhibition of Quadriceps Femoris in Patients after Reconstruction of Anterior Cruciate Ligament: a Protocol for a Randomized Controlled Trial. Journal of Acupuncture and Meridian Studies. 16: 193-202.
86. Velázquez, J., Ruíz, B., Rodriguez, D., Romero, C., López, D., Calvo, C. (2020). Efficacy of quadriceps vastus medialis dry needling in a rehabilitation protocol after surgical reconstruction of complete anterior cruciate ligament rupture.
87. Alaei, P., Nakhosin, N., Naghdi, S., Fakhari, Z., Komesh, S., Dommerholt, J. (2020). Dry Needling for Hamstring Flexibility: A Single-Blind Randomized Controlled Trial. Journal of Sport Rehabilitation. 30(3).
88. Nakhosin, N., Alaei, P., Naghdi, S., Fakhari, Z., Komesh, S., Dommerholt, J. (2018). Immediate Effects of Dry Needling as a Novel Strategy for Hamstring Flexibility: A Single Blinded Clinical Pilot Study. Journal of Sport Rehabilitation. 29: 1-23.
89. Kumagai, M., Sato, M., Akazawa, K. (2016). Effects of dry needling on myofascial pain syndrome in the pectineus muscle: A case report. Journal of Bodywork and Movement Therapies. 20(2): 348-352.
90. König, L., Mense, S. (2014). The effect of dry needling on pain and muscle stiffness in the adductor longus muscle: A case study. Journal of Bodywork and Movement Therapies. 18(1): 124-130.
91. López, M., Gallo, F. (2017). Efficacy of dry needling on the adductors in patients with groin pain. Fisioterapia. 39(1): 23-29.
92. Cecchini, M., Gonzalez, A. (2016). The effect of dry needling on myofascial pain syndrome in the adductor muscles: A randomized controlled trial. Pain Medicine. 17(12): 2284-2291.
93. Rahou, Y., Navarro, M.J., Gomez, G.F., Cleland, J.A., Lopez, I., Fernandez, C., Ortega, R., Plaza, G. (2020). Effects of trigger point dry needling for the treatment of knee pain syndromes: a systematic review and meta-analysis. J.Clin. Med. 9.

94.- Ughreja, R.A., Prem, V. (2021). Efficacy of dry needling techniques in patients with knee osteoarthritis: a systematic review and meta-analysis. J. Bodyw. Mov. Ther. 27: 328-338.
95.- Mayoral, O., Salvat, I., Martin, M., Martin, S., Santiago, J., Cotarelo, J., et al. (2013). Efficacy of myofascial trigger point dry needling in the prevention of pain after total knee arthroplasty: a randomized, double-blinded, placebo-controlled trial. Evid Based Complement Alternat Med.
96.- James, S.L., Ali, K., Pocock, C., Robertson, C., Walter, J., Bell, J., et al. (2007). Ultrasound guided dry needling and autologous blood injection for patellar tendinosis. British Journal of Sports Medicine. 41(8):518-21
97.- Velázquez, J., Sánchez, Z., Campón, A., Chekroun, A., Baraja, L. (2022). Comparative Study of the Efficacy of Hyaluronic Acid, Dry Needling and Combined Treatment in Patellar Osteoarthritis Single Blind Randomized Clinical Trial. International Journal of Environmental Research and Public Health (IJERPH). 19(7).
98. Reza, M., Kordi, A., Rahimi, M., Abdollahian, N. (2021). Myofascial Pain and Treatment Dry needling trigger points around knee and hip joints improves function in patients with mild to moderate knee osteoarthritis. Journal of Bodywork and Movement Therapies. 27: 597-604.
99. Espejo, L., Gacimartín, A., Pérez, M.R., Cardero, M.A., De la cruz, B., Albornoz, M. (2014). Effects on adverse neural tension measured by Slump test after myofascial trigger point dry needling of the gastrocnemius muscle. Physiotherapy. 36(3): 127-134.
100. Lucena, D., Luque, C., Valencia, J., Garcia, C. (2022). Effectiveness of Dry Needling of Myofascial Trigger Points in the Triceps Surae Muscles: Systematic Review. Healthcare. 10(10): 1862.
101. Mullins, J., Nitz, A., Hoch, M. (2019). Dry needling equilibration theory: A mechanistic explanation for enhancing sensorimotor function in individuals with chronic ankle instability. Physiotherapy Theory and Practice. 37: 1-10.

102. Salemi, P., Hosseini, M., Daryabor, A., Fereydounnia, S., Smith, J. (2024). Trigger Point Dry Needling to Reduce Pain and Improve Function and Postural Control in People With Ankle Sprain: A Systematic Review and Meta-Analysis. Journal of Chiropractic Medicine.

103. Singh, A., Wadhwani, N., Sharma, M. (2024). Short-term effectiveness of dry needling on pain and ankle range of motion in athletes with medial tibial stress syndrome- a randomized control trial. The Journal of manual and manipulative therapy. 1-7.

104. Mullins, J., Hoch, M., Kosik, K., Heebner, N., Gribble, P., Westgate, P., Nitz, A. (2020). Effect of Dry Needling on Spinal Reflex Excitability and Postural Control in Individuals With Chronic Ankle Instability. Journal of Manipulative and Physiological Therapeutics. 44.

105. He, C., Ma, H. (2017). Efficacy of trigger point dry needling for plantar heel pain: a meta-analysis of seven randomized controlled trials. J. Pain Res. 10 :1933-1942.

106. Llurda, L., Labata, N., Meca, T., Navarro, M.J, Cleland, J.A., Fernandez, C., Perez, A. (2021). Is dry needling effective for the treatment of plantar heel pain or plantar fasciitis? A systematic review and updated meta-analysis. Pain Med. 22 :1630-1641.

107. Cotchett, M.P., Munteanu, S.E., Landorf, K.B. (2014). Effectiveness of trigger point dry needling for plantar heel pain: a randomized controlled trial. Phys Ther. 94: 1083-94.

108. Eftekhar, B, Babaei, A, Zeinolabedinzadeh, V. (2012). Evaluation of dry needling in patients with chronic heel pain due to plantar fasciitis. Foot (Edinb). 1-5.

109. Salehi, S., Shadmehr, A., Olyaei, G., Bashardoust, S. (2019). Effectiveness of dry Needling for the management of plantar fasciitis: A review Study. Journal of modern rehabilitation. 13(1).

110. Behnam, A., Mahyar, S., Ezzati, K., Rad, S.M. (2014). The use of dry needling and myofascial meridians in a case of plantar fas-ciitis. Journal of Chiropractic Medicine. 13(1): 43-8.

111. El Mallah, R., Elattar, E.A., Zidan, H.F. (2017). Platelet-rich plasma versus dry needling of myofascial meridian trigger points in the treatment of plantar fasciitis. Egyptian Rheumatology and Rehabilitation.44(2): 58.

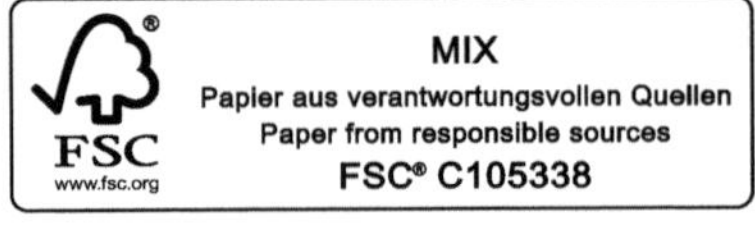

Printed by Books on Demand GmbH, Norderstedt / Germany